Fundamental aspects of gynaecology

Note

Health care practice and knowledge are constantly changing and developing as new research and treatments, changes in procedures, drugs and equipment become available.

The author and publishers have, as far as is possible, taken care to confirm that the information complies with the latest standards of practice and legislation.

Fundamental aspects of gynaecology

Sandra Johnson

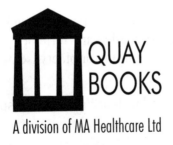

QUAY
BOOKS

A division of MA Healthcare Ltd

Quay Books Division, MA Healthcare Ltd, St Jude's Church, Dulwich Road, London SE24 0PB

British Library Cataloguing-in-Publication Data
A catalogue record is available for this book

ISBN 1 85642 274 7

Printed in the UK by Ashford Colour Press Ltd, Gosport, Hampshire

Contents

Foreword

The aim of this book is to present the reader with a current account of the more common gynaecological problems with which women can suffer and to offer nurses an insight into the medical, nursing, social and legal issues that surround many female reproductive tract anomalies.

Women and men have many anatomical and physiological commonalities and similar needs for the development of self concept, self esteem and self fulfilment. Many health needs correspond, in that both genders require a suitably balanced diet, safety and security in order to grow, and education to develop an ability to live effectively in an ever-advancing world.

The need to reproduce is an innate force common to all living organisms in order for the species to survive, but in all life forms this is sometimes undesirable due to genetic factors or hostile environmental conditions.

Some of these issues will be explored within the following chapters and, whilst answers to health problems cannot always be exact, it is anticipated that helpful information can be found here.

The book concentrates on gynaecological (science of women) issues, but certain aspects, particularly in relation to reproduction, necessarily involve paying attention to men's health.

An assumption is made that the reader has a reasonably good comprehension of the anatomy and physiology of the female reproductive tract and the influences upon it from pituitary and hypothalamic activity. However, there are numerous very readable texts that can be accessed in order to revise and become more familiar with the system, including Guyton and Hall (2000), Clancy and McVicar (2002) and Tortora and Grabowski (2003).

In selecting the aspects to be addressed, several factors were considered, for example epidemiological issues such as a general increase in the elderly population (see Chapter 7, which addresses stress urinary incontinence), the rise in sexual activity in adolescents (see Chapters 2 and 4, which discuss abortion and infections/infestations of the female reproductive tract), and women's desire to take more control over their own physiological processes (see Chapters 1 and 3, which include contemporaneous information relating to fertility and menopause).

In writing this book, it was recognised by the author that as the nursing profession is largely female dominated, many nurses, whether or not involved directly with gynaecological care, are likely to be approached by friends, family members, neighbours or women who feel that a nurse should be able to answer their personal questions and that this book would indeed offer the reader an insight into 'Fundamental Aspects' of gynaecology.

It is not a comprehensive account of all of the pathological conditions that can affect the female reproductive tract; rather, it is a useful resource book for both student and Registered nurses' reference when questions arise in relation to health education/promotion, women's decision-making with respect to treatments available and legal issues that may need to be addressed.

Dr Ricky Autar
RGN, RMN, Dip Nursing (Lond), Cert Ed, RNT, B.Hons, MSc, PhD
Principal Lecturer
Head of Adult Division
School of Nursing and Midwifery
De Montfort University
Leicester
UK

References

Clancy, J and McVicar, A (2002) *Physiology and Anatomy*. Arnold, London

Guyton, A C and Hall, J E (2000) *Structure and Function of the Body*. W B Saunders, Philadelphia

Tortora, G J and Grabowski, S R (2003) *Principles of Anatomy and Physiology*. John Wiley, Massachusetts

Acknowledgements

I would like to thank my colleagues at De Montfort University for their help and encouragement with the completion of this book, especially John Fowler, who initiated the process, and Penny Tremayne, who continually rushed into my office, interrupting my thought processes with new ideas and enthusiasms – a lovely person to whom I owe a debt of gratitude.

I would also like to thank Dr Ricky Autar, with whom I have spent a great deal of my professional life at De Montfort University, and who has been very supportive throughout.

The most sustaining and patient person, who encouraged me to keep writing until the early hours of many mornings, therefore having to cook his own dinners and breakfasts – my husband – I cannot thank enough.

Sandra Johnson
Senior Lecturer in Nursing
De Montfort University
Leicester
UK

CHAPTER I

Fertility, infertility and unwanted fertility

Introduction

Fertility, conception, 'misconception', non-conception and contraception are words full of humour, joy, relief, dismay and devastation to many women and their partners, with families, friends, culture and religion all playing their part in affecting these emotions.

This chapter will address normal fertility and planning pregnancy, as well as some problems that may arise during a pregnancy. Some aspects of minor difficulties that couples wanting to have children might encounter, and how these may be overcome without resorting to medical intervention, will be presented and the problems of couples who appear unaccountably to be unable to reproduce together without medical intervention will be discussed.

The chapter will also offer guidance regarding the avoidance of pregnancy when couples feel that parenthood is inappropriate or unwanted.

It would be useful for the reader to have a definitive understanding of the following:

◇ Fertility
◇ Subfertility
◇ Infertility

◇ Menstrual cycle
  – Pre-ovulatory stage
  – Ovulatory phase
  – Post-ovulatory stage
◇ Conception
◇ Contraception
◇ AID (vs. AIDS)
◇ IVF
◇ GIFT

These will all, however, be explained within the text.

Fertility

A couple is said to be 'fertile' if conception has been achieved within 12 months of unprotected sexual intercourse (Pollard 1994). Healthy pregnancies depend upon the pre-pregnancy health of both parents – the healthier the parents, the fewer problems are likely to be encountered by the neonate.

Normal pregnancy is achieved by a male having unprotected sexual intercourse with a female during the ovulatory phase of the menstrual cycle, which is usually 14 days in a 28-day cycle. Spermatozoa enter the cervical canal, travel through the uterine cavity and along the fallopian tubes, meeting with the ovum, usually at the ampulla (expanded section) of the tube. Normally only the fittest sperm are able to survive this rigorous journey, and therefore natural selection operates to maximise the health of the offspring.

Mature ova are released by alternate ovaries at the rate of one per month, so whilst several million sperms may be present in the average 5 ml of ejaculated seminal fluid, many will not survive the cervical/uterine/fallopian route, and of those that do, at least 50% will enter the tube that contains no ovum.

The fertilised ovum migrates down the fallopian tube to the uterus, whose endometrial lining has been prepared by oestrogen to receive it, and implants into this thickened tissue usually within seven days post-ovulation (Belfield 1999).

Once implantation has taken place the fertilised ovum (embryo) produces human chorionic gonadotrophin (hCG) which influences the ovary to maintain the corpus luteum. In the non-pregnant state, the corpus luteum produces progesterone in a large amount just after ovulation, but this gradually diminishes until menstruation occurs. In the pregnant state, however, the hCG enables the corpus luteum to continue progesterone production, which sustains the growing embryo during pregnancy.

Obviously a woman will produce many ovaduring reproductive life, the majority of which will not be fertilised, and some of those that are will not successfully implant into the endometrium or will develop growth failure and be reabsorbed in the early days, with the woman being unaware of a possible conception. Some may fail to develop properly and will be expelled and experienced as a heavy menstrual period. For these reasons, pregnancy legally 'begins' at implantation of the fertilised ovum into the endometrium (Belfield 1999).

Following a successful implantation and persistence of the corpus luteum, no menstruation occurs on the '28th' day of the cycle, and it does not reoccur until after the birth of the child. Ova are not released during pregnancy. Whilst menstrual absence following unprotected sexual intercourse is often indicative of pregnancy, there are many other reasons for amenorrhoea or delayed menstruation: illness, stress, antibiotic therapy, cortisone, shift work and excessive alcohol intake, for example (Chubb and Knight 1992).

The developing embryo has two membranes that cover and protect it. The outer is known as the chorion and the membrane closest to the embryo is the amnion. From the chorionic layer, finger-like projections develop (chorionic villi) which attach to the uterine wall and move nutrients from the maternal blood to the embryo. Later during pregnancy this immature blood supply system forms the placenta, which is the nutritional source for the remainder of the foetus's development.

The developing foetus is immersed in the amniotic sac surrounded by fluid (amniotic fluid) and connected to the placenta by the umbilical cord. The cord is a transport mechanism for the foetal receipt of nutrients and return of waste products from and to the mother. The placenta is also an endocrine gland that produces oestrogen, progesterone and hCG. The placenta takes over from the ovarian production of these hormones and increases blood levels in the mother to sustain the foetal development. The high levels of hCG circulating in the bloodstream following placenta formation lead to detectable levels of the hormone excreted in the urine – which forms the basis of pregnancy testing.

Many pregnancy self-testing kits are available over the counter from high street chemists, and whilst most are reliable, women should not have complete faith in them, as false negative and false positive results have been reported (Mack and Tucker 1996) which may raise or dash hopes unnecessarily. Blood test hCG levels of above 10 international units/litre (iu/l) and urine levels of above 25 iu/l are generally considered to be positive signs of pregnancy.

Maternal physiological changes during pregnancy

A woman's normal physiological processes need assistance to cope with the extra load of pregnancy. Because homoeostatic regulation during this time is set at a new level, adaptive maternal changes of cardiovascular function and metabolism occur in order to support the growth and development of the growing foetus. The placenta, being an additional hormone source once developed, supplements essential neuro-endocrine and immunological systems. It exchanges heat, nutrients and waste products between mother and child, but also allows transmission of viruses that can cause death *in utero* or serious life-challenging situations for the neonate.

These viruses include the Human Immunodeficiency Virus (HIV), the organism responsible Acquired Immune Deficiency Syndrome (AIDS), which is potentially fatal, and the rubella virus, which causes 'German Measles' and can damage the foetal heart, lungs, eyes ears and brain. These conditions, along with others are always investigated via blood tests early in a pregnant mother's antenatal situation so that protective measures may be discussed.

The placenta cannot discriminate between a toxin and a nutrient and factors such as tobacco smoke will affect the transport of nutrients and oxygen, leaving the foetus at risk of starvation of these life essentials. Pollard (1994) discusses the trend in Western societies of a general lowering incidence of cigarette smoking population-wide, but an increase in smoking among younger women of childbearing age. Cigarette smoke contains numerous hazardous compounds that may cause harm to the developing foetus by inducing intra-uterine hypoxia and causing uterine vasoconstriction, which further decreases placental perfusion and oxygen availability. Currently there are about 13 million adults who smoke in the UK, some of whom are pregnant, but even if the latter do not smoke themselves, their offspring are at risk if the mother is exposed to passive smoking (Action on Smoking and Health 2001).

Soon after implantation (within about 28 days) the foetal heart and circulatory system becomes the first to function. The portion of the uterus that contains the chorionic villi, known as the decidua basalis, is the maternal part, and this and the foetal portion, or chorion frondosum, function concurrently as the placenta, promoting the effective exchange of nutrients and gases. Thus any placental trauma or growth retardation will affect foetal development (Ahmed *et al* 1992). The mother's cardiac output increases by about 40% – from 5 litres per minute to 7 litres per minute – which is achieved by an increased heart beat and increased stroke volume.

These, together with expanded blood cell and plasma volumes, provide an extra force to meet the heightened demand of tissues for nutrients during pregnancy. Vascular resistance is reduced, however, to prevent dangerous hypertension, and extra metabolic heat generated by the foetus is convected away from the mother by means of increased peripheral circulation of hands, arms and legs. Blood loss of, on average, 500 ml during vaginal delivery is countered by the expanded blood volume that occurs during pregnancy.

Towards the end of pregnancy, respiratory efficiency is increased by about 30%, brought about by a rise in tidal volume, equalling approximately an extra 3 litres per minute (Clancy and McVicar 2002). The haemoglobin concentration of foetal blood is approximately 50% greater than the maternal status, which affords an increased amount of oxygen to be transported to the foetus. At delivery, foetal haemoglobin is about 17 g/dl, which is well above the usual adult concentration of 11–12 g/dl. However, due to haemolysis of damaged or worn out erythrocytes postnatally, the foetal haemoglobin reduces to the adult concentration within just a few weeks. Iron from these haemolysed cells is stored in the foetal liver to compensate for the fact that the milk-fed neonate receives a low iron diet of 1–2 mg/l, which is insufficient to sustain the neonatal need for haemopoiesis.

During pregnancy, the efficiency with which the mother's food intake is converted into usable energy will vary with individual eating habits, type, calorific content and the proportion of protein, fat and carbohydrate that the food contains, but additional energy requirements during pregnancy involve (Whyte and Donaldson 1999):

◇ increased food ingestion
◇ increased utilisation of maternal food stores
◇ increased absorption of energy
◇ decreased general energy output
◇ decreased resting metabolic rate

Parturition (approximately 40 weeks gestation)

Immediately before birth, endocrine activity between mother, foetus and placenta combines to stimulate and maintain parturition, or birth of the infant. Oestrogens, progesterone, relaxin, oxytocin, prostaglandins, catecholamines, cortisol and endorphins interact to produce uterine contractions, provide a degree of analgesia, maintain those myometrial contractions and ensure cervical widening to allow the foetal head to descend into the vagina.

The end result is the sequential maturing of an intercommunicating endocrine system between mother and foetus, which should normally result in the delivery of a healthy infant.

Lactation

Parturition triggers lactation. During pregnancy, growth and maturation of the lobules and alveoli of breast tissue proliferates under the influence of increased hormone levels, and by the third month of pregnancy there is a thick liquid secreted by the breast alveoli, stimulated by placental lactogen. However, true lactation (production and delivery of genuine breast milk) does not become possible until the third trimester.

During the first week after the baby is delivered, the breasts secrete a watery fluid – colostrum – which is rich in antibodies that are passed to the suckling infant to provide a degree of passive immunity during its early life. Soon after, the breasts secrete true breast milk that provides the neonate with all the nutrients required for normal growth and development. The volume of milk produced is influenced by the suckling action of the infant, the coordinated action of a number of hormones and the gradual progression of the infant to a solid diet. Prolactin is the main hormone, secreted by the pituitary gland, that controls breast milk production, but growth hormone, placental lactogen, and thyroid and adrenal corticoid hormones all have a specific part to play (Pollard 1994).

Due to the highly nutritive and immunological content of human maternal milk, breast feeding is to be encouraged, even if only for a short time. Nevertheless, milk volume and content deplete the mother's energy stores, and if for dietary or other reasons she has poor storage levels, breast feeding will deplete her nutritional reserves. This is particularly the case with calcium, as breast milk maintains a normal content of the mineral by drawing on the calcium reserves of the mother's bones and teeth, which may have implications for the development of osteoporosis in later life (Ben-Jonathan *et al* 1991).

Many maternally ingested drugs will pass into breast milk, as will pathogenic organisms, having a subsequent effect upon the suckling infant. It has become an ironic fact that women in underdeveloped countries who have been encouraged to breast feed their children to avoid expensive 'exploitative' dried milk powder products have seen their young die from AIDS as a result of HIV infection passing to them via maternal breast milk (Whittaker 2004).

Role of the nurse/midwife

The most effective measures in ensuring healthy pregnancy, childbirth and subsequent early neonatal growth and development lie in effective education of both parents.

A pre-pregnancy plan can be obtained from the Family Planning Information Service, 27–35 Mortimer Street, London, W1N 7RJ, local Family Planning clinics and general practitioner surgeries and health centres.

The knowledgeable nurse/midwife will be able to explain the problems posed by poor pre-pregnancy maternal nutrition – a low birth-weight baby that is slow to grow and late in achieving developmental milestones, which may disadvantage a child's future learning abilities.

The avoidance of noxious substances can be included in discussions of a general nature between the nurse's/midwife's family, friends and acquaintances. Providing the health care worker can explain the hazards associated with such issues as maternal exposure to rubella prior to conception, the effects of increasing age, a rapid succession of pregnancies and a high parity rate, women may well be encouraged to consider their pre-conceptual lifestyle and make adjustments accordingly.

There are also risks that apply to the offspring of both potential parents, though the paternal situation is less well documented. Moderate to heavy paternal alcohol intake and cigarette smoking can cause sperm count reduction and sperm damage that can result in serious foetal abnormality.

Few potential parents wish knowingly to adversely affect their child's pre- or post-natal development, but may not fully realise the potential effects of noxious substances, nor that if both parents indulge in the substance use (e.g. smoking tobacco), then the risk to the infant's well-being is doubled (Whyte and Donaldson 1999).

Education regarding reproduction, contraception, pregnancy and the financial and personal implications of becoming a parent may help to reduce or eliminate some potential cases of infant growth retardation, and nurses and midwives are well placed to inform prospective parents of these issues.

Babies born at weights of 2500 g or under frequently require expensive neonatal care and may need further health and social care due to related disabling conditions. Pollard (1994) asserts that it is of national interest to assist the young and the poor, as these two groups are at greatest risk of delivering low birth-weight babies. Effective contraception methods are discussed with adolescents by school nurses, but this has not led to a decrease in teenage pregnancies; in fact, the UK has the highest percentage of such births in Europe (Andrews 1999).

In 2000, there were 98,000 conceptions amongst teenage girls in England and Wales. Of these, 8000 were to girls under 16 years. From this number, 61% proceeded to maternity and 39% to abortion. The number of conceptions to girls under 14 years was 400, of which 160 continued to maternity. These figures, quoted by National Statistics (2003), are more than 40% higher than the country with the next highest rate – Portugal – with Italy, Sweden and Denmark's teenage pregnancies being less than a quarter of the rate in England and Wales.

There are numerous ethical and moral arguments surrounding the issues of giving or withholding expensive treatment to potentially, but unnecessarily, handicapped foetuses. Pollard (1994) states that, in her view:

If a humane community judges that failure to provide life-preserving treatment to a needy new-born constitutes child neglect, then failure to make adequate preventive provisions to minimise the need for intervention at birth, likewise constitutes a failure in basic human rights. It is the children who are being punished by social neglect and ignorance.

Nurses and midwives, the majority being female, are frequently turned to by teenage girls for advice about pregnancy, abortion, contraception and social issues related to these topics, and must be in possession of contemporaneous facts and be able to offer empathic support during what, for many of these young people, will be a traumatic time, often resulting in long-term effects.

Fertility rates

Fertility patterns vary, and these variations inevitably influence family size and the age structure of the population generally. Following the two world wars during the 20th century, fertility rates peaked briefly and then again about 18–20 years later as the post-war babies reached sexual maturity and had their own children.

In the UK at the beginning of the 20th century there were about 115 live births per 1000 women in the reproductive range of 15–44 years, but this declined to an all-time low in 2000 of 55 live births per 1000 women of similar age. Although there is a high rate of teenage pregnancies, the general UK trend is towards later childbirth, with the average age of women at childbirth generally being 29.1 years (National Statistics 2003).

According to Womack (2003), who quotes from a focus group and survey research of 1500 adults, this is because:

Professional thirty-somethings want to enjoy the good life for longer.

The research suggested that many potential parents view children as:

mixed blessings with clear penalties, especially for women.

Conducted by the Institute of Public Policy Research, the report concluded that Britain's current birth rate of 1.64 children per female is only slightly higher than the European average of 1.53, and even China, which has a 'one child only' policy, maintains a fertility rate of 1.83. In Britain, 1 in 5 women are childless at 40 years of age and 1 in 4 of the respondents in their late 30s did not have children. Many women in their early 30s were delaying motherhood for financial reasons, assuming that the decision to become pregnant in their late 30s would still be their own.

Given the effects of ageing on reproductive tissue, the growing trend towards childlessness may be linked to women postponing pregnancy and hence experiencing difficulty in conceiving.

Economists suggest a gloomy economic future for this country if the current downward fertility rate continues, with just two employees contributing towards the costs of every pensioner compared with seven in 1950 (Womack 2003).

Whilst most conceptions progress to a normal pregnancy and delivery, sadly there are many problems that can affect mother or foetus or both. Some are reversible, treatable or containable, but unhappily, some result in death of the foetus. Even today, when maternal death rates are considered to be very low, this is still a reality that nurses and midwives may encounter, and ectopic pregnancy is a potentially fatal condition for a pregnant woman.

Ectopic pregnancy

This is a relatively common condition which affects about 1 in 90 pregnancies and accounts for over 20,000 emergency hospital admissions annually (Royal College of Obstetricians and Gynaecologists (RCOG) 2002). Moreover, Tay (2000) reports that the increasing incidence of pelvic inflammatory disease and chlamydial infection appears to be responsible for the increasing number of ectopic pregnancies.

Ascending sexually introduced pathogens cause inflammation of the fallopian tube lining, whose specialised ciliated epithelial cells are damaged and hence the fertilised ovum (embryo) is not effectively transported to the uterine cavity. It becomes embedded in the tubal wall and continues to grow as it would, had normal implantation in the endometrium taken place. The fallopian tube cannot continue to expand to accommodate the growing embryo and stretching of its wall causes bleeding (which is usually, but not always revealed per vagina) and abdominal pain.

If misdiagnosis occurs at this time – and the Ectopic Pregnancy Trust (2004) (`http://www.ectopic.org.uk/`) states that this is not uncommon – the tube can rupture, causing severe internal bleeding, rapidly induced shock and death. According to Abbott (2004), death from misdiagnosed ectopic pregnancy is

> The third biggest killer of pregnant women in the UK after thromboembolism and hypertension.

On average, five such deaths amongst pregnant women occur annually, which is an avoidable tragedy. Jain (1988) asserts that an intrauterine pregnancy can be detected by transvaginal scanning from four weeks and according to Stabile (1996) a gestational sac is always seen when hCG levels rise above 30 iu/l.

It is therefore unacceptable that such deaths occur, and allegations of breach of medical duty could be avoided if standard guidelines issued by the RCOG (2002) were adhered to diligently.

Sites of ectopic pregnancy

From least to most common (Winston 1994; see Figure 1.1):

◇ Occasionally the ovum, having been released from the ovary, is not ensnared by the fimbriated end of the fallopian tube and may be fertilised within the pelvic cavity. There have been a few reported cases of successful pregnancies arising from pelvic fertilisation, but these are more likely to fail to progress due to inability to implant into pelvic organs (Ankum 2000). Statistics are thus difficult to assess.

◇ The embryo may successfully traverse the tube only to become trapped in the interstitial section of the tube, i.e. the wall of the uterus where tube and uterus meet. There is slightly more room for embryonic growth at this site, and therefore the point of diagnosis and potential rupture would be later than if the implantation occurs in a narrower portion of the fallopian tube. Rosevear (2002) reports that approximately 2% of ectopic pregnancies arise at this position.

◇ A slightly more common site of ectopic pregnancy (5%) is at the fimbrial end of the tube, where again, as there is greater potential for embryonic expansion, symptoms suggesting an ectopic preg-

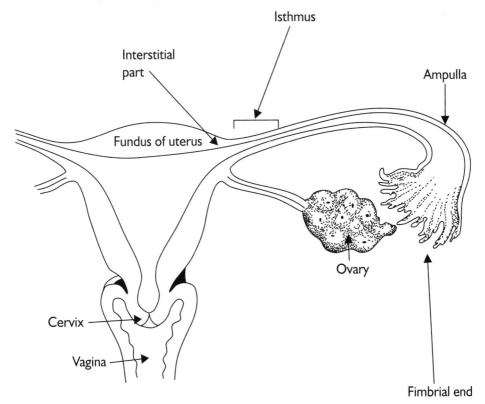

Figure 1.1: *Sites of ectopic pregnancy.*

nancy may be a little later than would be expected were it sited in a narrower tubal section.

◇ The third most common site is at the isthmus – 12%.
◇ Most commonly, about 80% of all ectopic pregnancies arising in the ampulla.

Predisposing factors to ectopic pregnancy

Factors that may lead to ectopic pregnancy are (Stabile 1996):

◇ Trauma to the fallopian tubes that has caused narrowing or obstruction that impedes the progress of the embryo, to the degree that it begins to implant into the tubal wall.
◇ Use of an intrauterine contraceptive device (IUCD). These are designed to prevent implantation in the uterus, but may occasionally lead to early implantation in the tube.
◇ Previous pelvic inflammatory disease, which may leave adhesions that constrict the tube (e.g. appendicitis).
◇ Sexually transmitted disease, in particular chlamydia, which has increased by 103% in the five years from 1997–2002 to 82,206 reported cases (Hartley 2004), although gonorrhoea is also becoming more common following a decline in past decades.
◇ Previous ectopic pregnancy, which may be due to one of the above factors.
◇ A previous history of infertility – particularly where *in vitro* fertilisation (IVF) has been instituted. In some women, following embryo transfer to the uterus the embryo migrates into the tube and continues its growth *in situ*.
◇ Following a previous Caesarean section. Since the incidence of delivery by this method is rising, women should be informed of risks for future pregnancies.
◇ Increasing maternal age – ectopic pregnancies are more common in women over 35 years than in younger women.
◇ Smoking tobacco appears to be implicated in ectopic pregnancy.

The signs and symptoms of ectopic pregnancy usually appear quite early after conception and the woman may not realise that she is pregnant, particularly if an IUCD has been inserted. Ectopic pregnancy is rare after the tenth week, so the symptoms that a woman suffers which may be suggestive of an ectopic pregnancy are more likely to be due to threatened or inevitable spontaneous abortion at that time (Winston 1994).

Once a woman begins to present with symptoms of an ectopic pregnancy, it is essential that she is investigated without delay to prevent unnecessary morbidity and potential death.

Common symptoms include:

◇ Abdominal pain, frequently unilateral but may be on the opposite side to the foetus (referred pain).
◇ Vaginal spotting or more heavy bleeding, although the blood is distinguishable from the normal menstrual flow by its darker colour and more watery consistency. Bleeding is not always apparent.
◇ Pain at the shoulder tip. This is 'referred' pain from internal bleeding, which irritates the phrenic nerve of the diaphragm and is referred along one of its several pathways to the thoracic apex.
◇ Possible dysuria/urgency of micturition and a feeling of increased pressure in the colon and rectum, inducing the bowel evacuation stimulus.

Acute symptoms are:

◇ Nausea, increased abdominal pain and rigidity
◇ Circulatory shock and collapse

Diagnosis, when undertaken early, is aimed at preserving fertility and reducing severe ill health. The foetus, unfortunately, cannot be rescued due to an interrupted blood supply. Diagnostic tests, if the woman is reasonably well, include an ultrasound scan and blood test for beta hCG levels to confirm pregnancy. If the blood test is positive, yet the scan shows no intrauterine contents, then it is likely that an ectopic pregnancy exists and needs to be further investigated to confirm or rule out its presence. Generally this involves further blood tests at 48-hour intervals, providing the woman remains sufficiently well. However, Tay (2000) argues that this method is unreliable and advocates laparoscopy to confirm diagnosis.

Early diagnosis offers the best chance of preserving fertility and may involve laparoscopy and suction removal of the embryo with minimal tubal damage. Alternatively, drug therapy, such as intramuscular methotrexate, or injected via laparoscopy and ultrasonography into the embryo, prevents its continued growth and the tissue is slowly absorbed into the woman's circulatory system. The RCOG (2002) recommends this approach in preference to laparotomy since the former aids a more rapid recovery for the woman, is more likely to preserve her future fertility and results in less morbidity.

According to Rosevear (2002) the success rate of 'expectant management', i.e. early diagnosis, methotrexate treatment and beta hCG blood level monitoring, is up to 70%. Alternative medical treatment to methotrexate involves prostaglandins or hyperosmolar glucose.

Surgical intervention for unruptured ectopic pregnancies is aimed at preservation of the fallopian tube and may be:

◇ Laparoscopic linear salpingotomy – the haemoperitoneum is accessible to the aspiration and suction/irrigation mechanism employed to evacuate the products of the ectopic pregnancy.
◇ Laparoscopic salpingectomy – indicated in approximately 10% of ectopic pregnancies. A small laparotomy incision may be necessary in order to perform the salpingectomy and removal of the pregnancy and manage any other coexisting gynaecological problem where possible. This method is usually necessary following ruptured ectopic pregnancy, where severe tubal damage and blood loss has occurred.

Role of the nurse

Nurses must understand the physiological and psychological distress that the patient is undergoing, and must provide support for her. Physical care relates to the individual needs of the woman and will include fundamental issues such as monitoring of vital signs, personal hygiene, food and fluid intake, pain management, elimination and the need for the woman to rest and sleep in order to recover from the traumatic experience. The patient's partner must not be forgotten, as the situation is likely to be a shared misery.

Psychologically, the nurse must be supportive but must not offer hope for the sustainment of the pregnancy where there is none.

The laparotomy approach means greater discomfort and risks for the patient and a prolonged hospitalisation. The necessity of avoiding hospital-acquired infections and other complications cannot be overemphasised, as these may all add to an already distressing situation.

Brown (1999), found that patients are frequently unhappy with information given to them by health care workers, and since it is mandatory for nurses and midwives to (Nursing and Midwifery Council (NMC) 2002b)

> ...act always in a manner as to promote and safeguard the interests of patients...

one aspect of a nurse's/midwife's role in this situation is to explain the signs and symptoms of a suspected ectopic pregnancy and its potential effects on future health and fertility, and also to alert the pregnant woman to the possibility of a ruptured ectopic pregnancy and its possible consequences.

According to Yao and Tulandi (1997), overall rates for subsequent uterine pregnancy after salpingotomy are about 50%, with about 12% of women having a further ectopic pregnancy. Following total or partial salpingectomy, they reported 38% of women conceiving an intrauterine pregnancy from a sample of 3584 patients, with just below 10% of these having a recurrent ectopic pregnancy.

Yao and Tulandi (1997) reported that with a history of two ectopic pregnancies, about 66% of future pregnancies will be ectopic, but up to 20% of those so affected will have subsequent uterine pregnancies.

Conclusion

For many women, the proof of their womanhood is to produce healthy babies at a time that is right for them and their partners, to raise those children in a responsible manner and to help them avoid or manage the many dangers and difficulties that life will inevitably pose.

For some parents, their own pre-pregnancy lifestyles can have negative effects on the developing foetus, sometimes through ignorance of the potential effects or, possibly, because addictive lifestyle habits are difficult to move away or completely abstain from.

Pregnancies are, for the majority of women, generally happy and uneventful with the outcome being the delivery of a healthy full-term baby (Winston 1994). However, there are a number of problems that can arise, and whilst most of these can be surmounted by modern medical, nursing and midwifery interventions, some will unfortunately result in unviable pregnancies.

One common problem, occurring in about 9% of pregnancies is that of the potentially life-threatening condition of ectopic pregnancy.

If this problem is diagnosed and treated early, future fertility problems can be minimised. However, the loss of a conception, together with emergency surgery, such as is required in a ruptured ectopic pregnancy, can have a hugely distressing impact upon a woman's psychological health and personal relationships, and may also decrease her future fertility by more than 50%.

Herman (1997) discusses the post-traumatic stress disorder symptoms of women who have suffered such personal losses, including nightmares, over-vigilance and depression. There is often a feeling of being 'tricked' and/or 'robbed' of a very special situation (Sizoo 2002).

As Abbott (2004) asserts:

Deaths from ectopic pregnancies should not still be occurring.

and calls for all health professionals to be aware of the problem, its signs, symptoms and potentialities. She also argues that health care workers should educate women and their partners, and be able to direct them to help sources such as the Ectopic Pregnancy Trust.

Infertility

This section addresses a variety of aspects relating to infertility, including definitions and statistical trends of fertility and infertility. It will also discuss some of the personal doubts and anxieties felt by infertile or subfertile couples and factors that predispose to these states. Investigations into the causes of infertility and possible options regarding treatment will also be addressed. Useful contact points for couples seeking guidance, advice or general information will be included.

Infertility in the UK is relatively common. Winston (1994) states that

At least 1 in 10 couples have a problem trying to conceive.

However, Rosevear (2002) argues that infertility rises with age, with 1 in 7 couples between 30 and 34 years old reporting difficulties, rising to 1 in 5 from 35 years to 40 and 1 in 4 for people over the age of 40 years.

Infertility is described (Te Velde *et al* 2000) as

The inability of a couple to conceive after twelve months of regular, unprotected sexual intercourse.

Many couples take several months to conceive, and about 17 in 20 do so within 12 months of trying, which increases to 19 in 20 after two years.

Of couples who discontinue contraception in order to conceive, only half will conceive within three months, but after two years of attempting to conceive about 95% of couples will have achieved their aim.

Winston's (1994) figures indicate that about 50% of all infertility is of female origin, 30% is male and in 20% of cases both male and female partners appear to contribute to the infertile state.

Infertility may be primary, where no conception has ever occurred before between the couple, or secondary, where a previous pregnancy has occurred but the couple is now experiencing difficulty with a subsequent conception. Infertility is becoming more common amongst couples who delay their family, and about 1 in 6 will seek assistance for their problems from their GP.

Greenhall and Vessey (1990) indicated that 3% of all women aged 25–44 years were involuntarily childless and 6% of women who had conceived were unable to have as many children that they would have liked. Collins *et al* (1995) found that up to 25% of all women who were attempting to conceive had an episode of subfertility and more than two spontaneous abortions or stillbirths during their reproductive lives.

In order to optimise the chances of conception, pre-conceptual preparation is helpful:

◇ Both partners should cease smoking as smoking adversely affects fertility (Hughes and Brennan 1996). It also increases the risk of spontaneous abortion and can cause foetal growth retardation.
◇ Women who are attempting conception should limit alcohol intake to 1 or 2 units per week (HEA 1996).
◇ Obesity should be managed, and Body Mass Index (BMI) – weight (kg)/height (m^2) – should be maintained within the normal range of 18.5 to 24.9. Under or overweight females may have an irregularity of ovulation that affects conception (Garrow 1991).
◇ Males should also limit their alcohol intake and, since hyperthermia can affect spermatogenesis, men should avoid wearing tight underwear and trousers (Mieusset and Bujan 1995).
◇ Folic acid 0.4 mg may be taken as a daily supplement and for the first three months of pregnancy to help prevent neural tube deficits.

Psychological aspects

Some couples who have difficulty in conceiving wait several years before seeking medical help, and when they do that first consultation can have a major impact and be intensely traumatic. Those who do not experience a sympathetic, understanding reception, with clear outlines of an investigation/treatment plan, are likely to undergo greater distress than that arising from their infertility.

Pressure from friends, parents and other relatives may bring about feelings of guilt, anger and grief, together with depression and loss of self esteem. The couple may feel resentment towards others who have children and especially towards women undergoing termination of pregnancy. Intimate and embarrassing personal questions by the medics trying to help the couple, may lead to problems with their sexual relationship or obsessional feelings of having to have sexual intercourse 'at the right time' (Winston 1994).

It is not unusual for the couple to go through a 'grieving process', only to find that the support given to people having suffered a bereavement is not forthcoming in their case. For some couples this destructive situation leads to dissolution of their relationship.

Investigations of infertility

Whilst there are many routine investigations and tests that can identify specific contributory causes, infertility can remain unexplained in up to 30% of couples, but that does not mean that infertility cannot successfully be overcome (HFEA 2003).

A history must be taken from both partners, to include details of sexual activity, followed by a pelvic examination to detect any anatomical abnormality that might be contributing to the infertile situation. Coital history is noted together with any drug therapy that might be interfering with fertility, e.g. sulphasalazine, nitrofurantoin (RCOG 1998). Exposure to environmental pollutants, e.g. lead, should also be assessed.

Investigations usually begin with assessing the most common causes:

◇ Ovulatory factors – up to 15%
◇ Pelvic factors (tubal obstruction, endometriosis, infections) – up to 40%

◇ Sperm factors – up to 40%
◇ Abnormal cervical mucus which obstructs sperm penetration – around 5%

Female investigations

The following investigations may be carried out for women:

◇ Thyroid function tests in women with signs/symptoms of over- or underactivity of the thyroid and those with irregular menstrual cycles.
◇ Prolactin levels in women with amenorrhoea or symptoms of raised prolactin levels such as galactorrhoea.
◇ For evidence of ovulation, Follicle Stimulating Hormone (FSH) and Lutenising Hormone (LH) levels should be monitored on days 3–5 of the cycle with oestradiol levels. If the oestradiol is high, it produces a negative feedback effect on FSH levels. High FSH levels suggest a poor response by the ovary to producing mature ova (Rosevear 2002).
◇ Serum progesterone levels taken on day 21 indicate ovulation if the result is over 20 iu/l.
◇ A hystero-salpingogram can detect tubal obstruction and offer information about the uterine cavity.
◇ Laparoscopy can enable pelvic evaluation such as detecting ovarian disease, endometriosis and scarring from pelvic inflammatory disease.
◇ Testing for *Chlamydia trachomatis* infection is essential, as the infection is very common and may be entirely responsible for the infertile situation. Any infection causes tissue inflammation and exudation and, if this occurs within the female reproductive tract, may be severe enough to obstruct the fallopian tubes. If screening for *Chlamydia trachomatis* proves positive, then both partners should be treated with appropriate antibiotics (Gilbert 1993).

Male investigations

The following investigation may be carried out for men:

◇ Semen analysis. Fischel *et al* (1993) published an enhanced list of criteria for normal semen characteristics, which include:
  - Volume per ejaculate – minimum of 2 ml
  - Sperm count of 20 million/ml minimum
  - At least 50% of sperm present must be actively motile
  - At least 30% of sperm present must be normal in shape and size
  - There should be fewer than 1 million white cells/ml present
  - A minimum of 75% of sperm should be viable

Treating the male

Laboratory indications of oligospermia (low sperm count) or azoospermia (absence of sperms in the seminal fluid specimen) should be treated with caution until at least two specimens have been tested at intervals, with both giving the same indication. A single sample showing abnormalities should not be viewed as 100% valid, since many factors can affect the sperm count temporarily.

In cases of primary testicular failure, such as that following cytotoxic chemotherapy and post-inflammatory mumps orchitis, there is no treatment to correct the azoospermia, but in cases of retrograde ejaculation, where sperm are pushed into the bladder (which may be due to an obstruction in the vas deferens) it is possible to obtain sperm from the epididymis which can be used in *in vitro* fertilisation (IVF) and intracytoplasmic sperm injection (Mack and Tucker 1996).

In some men infertility is caused by antisperm antibodies, which cause sperm to clump together and then have greater difficulty in penetrating the cervix.

Sperm 'washing' may increase the possibility of fertilisation via intrauterine insemination (IUI), although the technique does reduce the sperm count to 10%. Since at least 1 million sperms are required for fertilisation, this will not be an option for males with oligospermia. However, Fischel *et al* (1995) reported a pregnancy following the use of surgically retrieved immature sperm (spermatids), and research continues into the possibility of offering greater success of fertility with this technique.

Minor surgical intervention may be very helpful, particularly where a varicocoele exists, but in situations where identifiable defects of sperm transport involving the vas deferens are found, success rates vary, and reduce with the amount of time that the obstruction exists.

Belker *et al* (1991) found that, following reversal of vasectomy, a patency rate of 97% was achieved after a 3 year post-operative interval and led to a 76% pregnancy rate. But after 15 or more years, patency was reduced to 71% with a subsequent pregnancy rate of 30%.

Treating the female

Endometriosis

Endometriosis is commonly implicated in infertility and its exact cause is unknown. The endometrium grows along the fallopian tubes and may exit; endometrial cells may migrate to the pelvic organs and compromise fertility by distorting female anatomy from adhesions that form between bladder, uterus, rectum and ovaries. Surgical removal of endometrial deposits may be necessary if medical treatment using anti-oestrogen drugs fails to reverse the condition.

Danazol is a useful drug in this respect, and is successful in approximately 50% of women so affected. Women who do not respond to danazol or who have severe side effects may react more favourably to GnRH agonists such as nafarelin or buserelin, with a return to normal fertility following treatment (Mack and Tucker 1996). Endometriosis was implicated as the prime cause of infertility in almost 10% of women seeking IVF in 1992 (HFEA 1994).

Pelvic inflammatory disease

Pelvic inflammatory disease following surgery, the use of intrauterine contraceptive devices and infections (particularly chlamydia) is the cause of many cases of female infertility and may be amenable to medical or surgical intervention, depending upon the severity of the situation and the length of time that it has been present.

Healey *et al* (1994) reported rapidly increasing levels of infertility with repeated episodes of infection and advocated early treatment of any woman with a sexually transmitted disease in order to preserve fertility where possible.

Disorder of ovulation

Anovulatory infertility requires investigation to exclude any ovarian pathology such as polycystic ovary syndrome, which is often associated with obesity, acne, hirsutism and dysfunctional menstruation.

Side effects from some medicines, such as anti-inflammatory analgesics and cytotoxic therapeutic chemicals, can also adversely affect ovulation and their involvement should be established. Once pathological causes of anovulatory infertility have been investigated and excluded, chemical induction of ovulation can be instigated.

Clomiphene citrate is the initial drug of choice – it causes an upsurge of gonadotrophic-releasing hormone which stimulates the ovarian follicle (Balen 1997). It is given for 5 days on day 2 after the start of menstruation, and similarly if the woman has been treated for amenorrhoea with progesterone, and has an induced withdrawal bleed. Dosage commences at a low level of 25–50 mg and the woman is monitored for subsequent ovulation. If this occurs, then the dose is maintained at this level, but if there are no signs of ovulation the dose can be increased to 150 mg daily for 5 days (Rosevear 2002).

Oestrogen levels should be monitored, together with ultrasound scans to assess growth of the follicles and prevent multiple pregnancy, unless this risk has been discussed with and accepted by the woman being treated (Balen 1997).

For women who suffer severe side effects from clomiphene, such as nausea and vomiting and/or visual/balance disturbances, tamoxifen may be a preferable prescription. There is a small but significant link between clomiphene therapy and ovarian malignancy where the drug is used for more than 12 months (Rossing *et al* 1994).

The results of this therapy are pleasing in that nearly 85% of conceptions occur during the first three ovulatory cycles of treatment, although dosages often have to be adjusted to suit the individual woman.

There is up to an 8% risk of multiple pregnancy, from 6.9% twins to 0.13% quadruplets (Rosevear 2002), but she reports no difference in the incidence of congenital abnormalities (2.5%) between treated and untreated women, and the incidence of spontaneous abortion appears to be similar at approximately 15%.

Gonadotrophin therapy

This treatment, using recombinant Follicle Stimulating Hormone (FSH), may be indicated for women who have not ovulated in response to clomiphene therapy. After one year there is a cumulative live birth rate of 60%, but multiple pregnancies feature in up to a fifth of those and spontaneous abortions may occur in 30% of cases.

During treatment the woman must be monitored by ultrasound for follicular maturation and/or serum oestradiol levels, which will indicate an appropriate response, as hyperstimulation must be avoided. The addition of GnRH or buserelin/goserelin will allow for more accurate timing of ovulation and sexual intercourse or assisted conception techniques.

Ovarian drilling

The ovary may be punctured up to 10 times each which induces endocrine changes that may be effective for up to six years post-operatively, with the result of improved ovulation of up to 80% and over 50% pregnancies. Additionally, the chances of pregnancy in combination with

IVF following ovarian drilling are also increased. The surgery needs to be carried out with care to avoid the risks of adhesions, premature ovarian failure or hyperstimulation (which may be life-threatening).

The HFEA (1995) published the live birth rate figures achieved for the previous year for each licensed clinic for the first time, which enabled couples to make comparisons. These should be treated with caution, as there are a number of variables that affect choices of this nature. These include costs; few Health Authorities will fund treatment for infertility totally, although some Primary Care Trusts may contract with a particular clinic to partially fund treatment – so there may not be a choice if the NHS is paying towards the couple's investigation and therapy.

The couple needs to be aware of any extra costs on top of those quoted for the initial treatment programme. The cost of infertility treatment varies. Donor insemination treatment can cost between £100 and £500 and IVF from £800 to £3000 per treatment cycle (HFEA 2003). Considerations also include:

◇ The availability of a female doctor and patient support group
◇ Types of drugs used by the clinic and their possible side effects
◇ Waiting list for treatment/counselling/genetic screening
◇ Facilities for ovum collection and storage, and sperm donation and storage

Couples should be certain that they understand fully the implications of IVF before embarking on a treatment programme.

In vitro *fertilisation (IVF)*

This process is a clear and obvious example of medico-surgical progress during the last quarter of the 20th century. In 1978 the first child (Louise Brown) was born after IVF was developed by Steptoe and Edwards (1978), following two years of investigation and treatment of Louise's mother and nine years of infertility. Since then, around 70,000 births from IVF therapy have happened in this country and its success has led to many other surgical/medical interventions in an attempt to resolve infertility (Radcliffe 2003).

A major role for the nurse has become apparent which has developed from being the initial 'chaperone' to being the person who delivers most of the care involved in the IVF programme. Nurses now assess clients and discuss treatment processes, perform venepuncture, undertake scans and teach partners to carry out injection procedures, and many clinic nurses are involved with ovum retrieval and embryo transfer. Allanach (2003) states that:

> Nurses make a vital contribution to the assisted conception team, whether it is because of the communication, support and co-ordination they provide, or because of the more technical interventions.

Practice nurses are also involved in assisting couples who are unable to perform injections either on themselves or on each other. Fleming (2003) reports on the hugely successful results that the HFEA (2003) published in relation to the Assisted Conception Unit at the University College Hospital, London, of 39.1% success rate in women across the age range generally and 45.4% in women under 38 years. Fleming sees her nursing role as one of coordinator of the assessment, reporting of results and counselling situations, and confesses to experiencing the joys and disappointments of couples with them.

The main influential factor affecting the outcome of an IVF programme is the woman's age. With increasing age, spontaneous abortion, chromosome defects such as Trisomy 21 (Down's Syndrome) and follicular degeneration are more common. For those women whose infertility is secondary, i.e. have had a previous pregnancy, the chances of a successful IVF pregnancy are greater than for those with primary infertility (HFEA 2003).

The HFEA (2003) published national IVF results for the year 2000–2001 indicating that:

◇ 23,737 women received IVF treatment
◇ 4,621 single births resulted
◇ 1,579 twins were born

◇ 109 triplets resulted
◇ 2,810 cycles were abandoned
◇ 465 live births resulted from 1,972 donated sperms or ova

The HFEA has been involved in collecting data from clinics about treatments and the results of these, and in giving advice and consideration in respect of ethical issues relating to infertility. In 2001, the HFEA directed that only two embryos could be implanted into the uterus to avoid the high rate of multiple births following many assisted conception techniques. Sex selection is currently being debated, as is the testing of embryos for genetic disorders prior to implantation.

In 2002 the HFEA was granted more funds to extend its role as inspector of clinics after a much-publicised case of a Northern centre's white female client's delivery of a mixed-race child, due to an error of ovum/sperm mixing. Her egg had been fertilised by sperm that was not that of her partner.

This is probably another area for expansion of the nurse's role, as nursing work relates totally to the experience of patients.

The IVF technique

Exactly 35 hours following an injection of hCG, ova are collected and placed into a suitable medium and supplemented with a protein source. Washed sperm are added to the ova at the concentration of 50,000 per ovum and, after about 18 hours have elapsed, the eggs are microscopically inspected for signs of fertilisation. This is confirmed if two pro-nuclei, containing between them the full human genetic complement, are identifiable. The embryo begins dividing, and on days 2–3 the embryo(s) are transferred into the uterus to enable implantation. The surgeon will look for maximum success by transferring embryo(s) with even-sized cells and granular cytoplasm. The embryo(s) should develop according to a fairly rigid timescale.

Freezing of embryos and sperm

At the point where pro-nuclei are identified, embryos may be frozen for future use. Although embryos may be frozen at other stages, the process is most successful at the pro-nuclei position. Damage to cells during freezing is common, and needs to be avoided by a process of carefully controlled, systematic manoeuvres and computer monitoring. Embryos are then stored in liquid nitrogen at −196 °C for up to a decade, when the process then has to be reversed.

Rosevear (2002) states that:

> Sperm are a lot sturdier than embryos

and when collected, are mixed with an equal quantity of preservation medium. Although some sperm are lost during the freeze–thaw process, she argues that generally 40% of motile sperm will remain viable through the process.

All of the above suggests that IVF is very labour-intensive and costly, which has meant that many Health Authorities have withdrawn funding from what might be seen as 'not an illness requiring medical intervention' and more of a demand to the right of parenthood.

Debate has raged over the so-called 'postcode lottery' (Murdoch 2003), where women living on the opposite side of the same street are granted or denied NHS support for infertility treatment. However, the National Institute for Clinical Excellence (NICE) (2003) published guidelines in August 2003 relating to the proposal of free IVF treatment for women aged between 23 and 39 years and these will become reality by April 2005. This means that couples (Reid 2004):

> ... in which the woman is aged between 23 to 39 years and have been trying for a baby for 2 years, will be offered at least 1 free cycle of IVF treatment

The government did not, however, implement the full NICE recommendations – 'infertile couples should be offered 3 cycles by the NHS', despite the fact that couples are twice as likely to have a successful pregnancy with three treatments rather than one, but it expected to work towards that goal. The government also stated that priority would be given to:

> couples who did not have any children living with them.

Artificial insemination (AI) and intra-uterine insemination (IUI)

Artificial insemination may be the treatment of choice to overcome hostile female cervical mucus, male impotence and premature ejaculation, or where anatomical abnormalities cannot be effectively corrected to the degree where natural conception is achievable. AI introduces sperm directly into the cervix via the vagina, and IUI is a similar procedure, but where semen is prepared in the laboratory in order to maximise sperm potential, and usually involves stimulation of the woman's ovaries.

Sperm donations are constantly in demand by Assisted Conception Units, who appeal to healthy males between the ages of 18 to 40 years, when sperm are usually of good, fertile quality.

Sperm donations are required:

◈ for couples where the male has oligospermia or azoospermia
◈ for couples who wish to prevent the transmission of a genetic condition
◈ for lesbian couples who wish to have children

Donors are usually paid a small amount plus expenses, and may donate at specified intervals for up to 6 months. Sperm is 'quarantined' for 6 months, after which donors are requested to return for HIV clearance. Sperm is stored by number not name, but the donor's characteristics, such as ethnic group, height, eye and hair colour, build and even general interests are documented so that couples requesting donor sperm can expect a relatively close match (Burns 2003).

Legal issues

Whilst assisted conception techniques do allow couples who cannot have their own children to conceive, there are legal implications that have to be considered. The Human Fertilisation and Embryology Act 1990 (HFEA Act) which became effective on 1 August 1991, sets out a legal framework that attempts to protect the interests of all concerned. Nurses engaged in working in the area of infertility should be aware of the Act and its implications so that potential donors' and parents' questions can be answered and anxieties allayed.

Factors addressed by the Act include:

◇ Parenthood: the woman receiving treatment and her co-treated partner will be legal parents. Where the woman treated has no male partner/husband, the resulting child will have no legal father.
◇ The sperm donor: he has no legal relationship, rights over or obligations towards the child born by sperm donation. Equally, the child has no rights over or obligations to the donor.
◇ Information-giving: donor characteristics, as previously stated, are required to provide a closely matched offspring to infertile couples, but the donor's name may not be disclosed. However, the HFEA has, under the Act, a legal duty to inform those adults who ask, whether or not they were born as a result of sperm/ovum donation. Persons of 16 years or over are entitled under the Act to know if they might be related (as a result of being born by this method) to someone whom they wish to marry. The information to satisfy the enquiry does not necessitate revealing the donor's name.
◇ Consent: donors must give written consent to the use and storage of sperm/ova and any embryos produced from them. This includes use for treatment and/or research. Donors may attach conditions, but if these are very harsh they may find that the clinic does not accept the donation.
◇ Counselling: there is a legal obligation for clinics to offer counselling to men and women prior to sperm/ova donation, although donors do not have to take advantage of the service.

For further information see the National Gamete Donation Trust/Donor Conception network and HFEA details at the end of this chapter.

Gamete Intrafallopian Transfer (GIFT)

As with IVF, it might be necessary to stimulate the ovaries to provide optimum ova for mixing with sperm. The mixed ovum/sperm solution is then transferred into the fallopian tube prior to fertilisation. The HFEA will only licence GIFT when donated gametes are utilised.

Intracytoplasmic Sperm Injection (ICSI)

This involves the injection of a single sperm directly into the ovum and is useful when sperms have had to be surgically extracted from the testis. In some men, the absence or obstruction of the vas deferens may mean that, although the testes are producing sperms, they cannot proceed on their normal ejaculatory journey via the vasa for deposition at the cervix. Sperms then need to be surgically retrieved from the epididymis or testis. The ISCI process is undertaken in the laboratory as for IVF, and similarly fertilisation is considered effective when two pro-nuclei are seen under the microscope. Rosevear (2002) claims that:

> Delivery rates vary from 22%–30% per treatment cycle.

But she notes that there are double the rates of sex chromosome aberrations in comparison to those children who have been born without ICSI.

Tubal surgery

Whilst IVF has conquered many of the problems of fallopian tube disease, there remains a place for surgical intervention in some women. The HFEA (2003) argues that surgery may be appropriate, depending upon the extent of tubal damage (usually resulting from pelvic inflammatory disease, endometriosis or congenital abnormalities), and if successful, may fully restore fertility

Surrogacy

This is the commissioning of a fertile woman to have a pregnancy on behalf of an absolutely infertile woman, e.g. where there is absence of the uterus.

The infertile woman is usually given drugs to stimulate oocyte maturation, which are then collected and fertilised by her partner's sperm.

These may then be frozen for implantation into the surrogate mother at a later date, or transferred at the usual time of 2–3 days after the ultrasound – directed follicle aspiration. Alternatively, the infertile woman's partner's sperm may inseminate the surrogate mother.

A contentious issue, surrogacy first came to public awareness in 1982 when Kim Cotton was paid by an infertile couple to proceed with a pregnancy effected by the infertile woman's partner's sperm. At the time, there was no legislation relating to surrogacy; therefore Ms Cotton was not breaking the law. The situation, however, raised considerable public debate, including:

◇ Should women be paid for such a 'service'?
◇ Who is the legal mother of the child?
◇ How will the surrogate mother be affected by the handing over of the baby that she has carried for nine months?
◇ What is the situation should the surrogate mother refuse to part with the neonate?
◇ What happens to the child if it has a congenital abnormality and the commissioning couple refuses to accept the child?
◇ Will the commissioning woman harbour feelings of guilt, as she is not the child's natural mother?
◇ How will the situation affect the midwifery team, whose role during pre- and postnatal care is to foster the bonding process between parents and child?

In view of these issues, Dame Mary Warnock was asked to present a report and recommendations to Parliament so that future such cases could be carefully controlled.

As a result, the UK law today makes it clear that:

◇ Surrogacy is legal, subject to conditions.
◇ No money other than 'reasonable expenses' should change hands.
◇ The individuals involved should decide what constitutes 'reasonable expenses'.
◇ Any agreements made in relation to the process are not legally binding – the intended parents can do little to secure their situation before the birth of the child.
◇ Following the birth, a 'Parent Responsibility Agreement' can be arranged between the surrogate mother and intended father which gives equal rights over the neonate (in certain cases), but after 6 weeks the intended parents can apply for a 'Parental Order' that gives them full rights over the child and discontinues any rights by the surrogate mother.
◇ It is illegal to advertise for surrogate mothers or for potential surrogate mothers to advertise their services.

On 4 August 2004, baby 'Marcus' was the 500th surrogate baby to be born via the organisation 'Childlessness Overcome Through Surrogacy' (COTS) (http://www.surrogacy.org.uk/), from whom further information can be obtained.

Aborted foetal cells and infertility

A further minefield to consider in the issue of infertility is the use of aborted foetal cells in research and assisted conception for infertile couples.

On the one hand, there are the views of Wilkie (2003) who argues:

The first thing to distinguish, is that ethically, we can experiment on human tissue, but should not experiment on human beings. Accordingly, it is perfectly ethical to proceed with any and all types of stem cell research, as long as this is human tissue, but it is completely unethical to do embryonic stem cell research, which of its very nature, necessitates the killing of a human embryo to obtain stem cells.

An argument linked to this treatment relates to the potential emotional trauma that a child born as a result of stem cell manipulation may suffer from when becoming aware of the facts.

An alternative argument, put forward by Payne (2003), is that, since infertility is almost always a distressing and traumatic experience, medical advancements of this nature should be greeted with optimism and enthusiasm rather than by moralising and holding back on beneficial treatments.

Undoubtedly, there must be some legislation to manage the situation in a way that is acceptable to the majority, and which is in general sympathetic towards involuntary childlessness.

The HFEA (2004) has recently recommended approval of human cloning for therapeutic purposes, but not to make baby clones. Further legislation is to be expected in order to identify clear parameters for this technique.

Conclusion

Infertility appears to be increasing in incidence and causes a great deal of anxiety, self-doubt and relationship trauma. The need for either partner to overcome their parentless state may become all-consuming, to the extent that positive aspects of life become buried in a trough of destruction and despair.

Whilst one or several of the methods described in this chapter may help a couple to overcome infertility, it remains the case that some are destined to remain childless despite the most medically advanced therapies available.

Nurses working in this field need to develop counselling skills in order to help couples work through their problems, but also to be aware of self-help groups that couples can join. There is much relief to be gained by couples so affected from the knowledge that their anguish is not unique and that support can be derived from others who are in similar circumstances.

Contraception

This section addresses the issue of unwanted fertility and includes:

◇ General information relating to reproductive health and sexual health services available to the public.

◇ Some legal and ethical aspects that nurses should consider when becoming involved with clients and their reproductive capacity, which include confidentiality and protection of young people.

◇ The description of types of contraceptive medication and devices available, statistics relating to their efficacy, and the advantages and disadvantages of their use.

◇ Male and female sterilisation and the role of the nurse in educating clients regarding contraceptive choices, together with the inclusion of useful addresses for further information.

There is a constant stream of information available to those wishing to plan their families according to their own circumstances. Sometimes, when this appears in the media, it is under 'shock' headlines which at best can be misleading and at worst frighteningly inaccurate. Although a variety of contraceptive measures are available in the UK, unplanned pregnancies do occur, either as a result of contraceptive failure or unprotected sexual intercourse.

Family planning and sexual health are important health education and public health issues, and were a key target of the Department of Health's (1992) health strategy:

> Planned parenthood provides benefits for the health of individuals, families and communities. Family planning services aim to promote this by providing access to contraception, sterilisation and advice on unplanned pregnancy. Additionally, education, counselling and health promotion can enable prospective parents to choose healthy lifestyles and increase the chances that their children will be both wanted and healthy. Delaying and spacing pregnancies, and limiting family size, contributes to the physical and mental health of mothers and children, and general family well-being.

The UK has, however, seen a steady increase in teenage pregnancies (Social Exclusion Unit 1999), which has been variously attributed to poor contraceptive knowledge, limited access to services provided in the locality and the increase in alcohol consumption.

The government issued a target that teenage pregnancies should be reduced by half by 2010 (DOH 1999), and encouraged nurses (in particular school nurses) to develop their role in order to contribute significantly to the government's desired objective.

School nurses are well placed to give information in a setting where teenagers are likely to be receptive, thus reducing the trauma involved in the termination of unwanted pregnancies and disrupted education, which leads to reduced employment prospects and a greater risk of living in poverty.

Nearly all Health Authorities have young people's services, and details can be obtained from the Family Planning Association's Contraceptive Education Service. The service provides information, help and support with personal relationship difficulties in addition to contraceptive measures. Most hospitals offer genito-urinary medicine clinics for people who are concerned that they may have contracted a sexually transmitted disease, and many now provide contraceptive services with trained family planning staff in attendance.

General practitioners also offer contraceptive facilities and many have nurse-led family planning clinics which offer a relaxed, informal setting which aims to make younger people less reluctant to attend for guidance and help.

Whenever contraceptive advice or treatment for younger people is discussed, several legal and professional issues are raised, discussed below.

Consent to treatment

The Family Law Reform Act (1969) states that consent is effective if the young person has reached the age of 16 years, and thus parental consent is not required.

There was some concern in medico-legal circles in 1985, when Mrs Victoria Gillick challenged the supply of contraception by GPs to her daughters, who were under that age. Following a protracted series of court cases, the High Court finally ruled in favour of the medical profession, with conditions that the 'Fraser Guidelines' be followed (Gillick v West and Wisbech Area HA and the DHSS 1985).

Fraser Guidelines

◇ That the young person is able to understand the advice and its associated moral, social and emotional implications
◇ That the doctor could not persuade the young person to inform the parents that contraceptive advice was being sought, nor allow that information to be revealed by the doctor
◇ That the young person is likely to begin, or is having/likely to have unprotected sexual relations, whether or not advice is given
◇ That, if the advice or treatment was withheld, then the young person's physical or mental health would be likely to suffer
◇ The young person's best interests would be served if contraceptive advice/treatment were given without parental consent.

The Children Act (1989) further supports the issues outlined above, and stresses parents' responsibilities in this respect. In this Act:

> Children under 16 may also be able to give, or refuse consent depending upon their capacity to understand the nature of the treatment

and that it is for the doctor to make the decision about the child's ability in this respect. The Nursing and Midwifery Council (NMC 2002a) also recognises this, by stating that parental consent for treatment is usually required, but that this does depend upon the age and level of understanding of the young person.

Confidentiality

The duty of confidentiality to anyone under 16 years is the same as that owed to any other person. It should be respected during either doctor or nurse consultation. Any breach of confidentiality by either must be justifiable to the General Medical Council and/or Nursing and Midwifery Council respectively.

Harm prevention

Nurses must also abide by the NMC Code of Professional Conduct (2002b), in respect of actions and omissions that may potentially harm a patient/client. Whilst most nurses would agree that encouraging young people to discuss their sexual health/contraceptive needs with informed professionals is acting in their best interests, if treatment is not forthcoming and a pregnancy results this could be deemed to be negligence.

Equally, nurses and doctors have a duty to follow child protection guidelines if they feel that the young person is being sexually abused or coerced into having undesirable sexual activity.

Contraceptive medicines and devices

Female

The range of contraceptive methods has extended considerably since the introduction of the combined oral contraceptive pill during the 1960s. Research and development continued, and since the 1990s technology has meant the availability of a choice of very effective methods to prevent pregnancy. Most couples wishing to do so should be able to select a contraceptive to suit their individual needs.

Andrews (2000) noted that although over 70% of sexually active women in this country were making use of some form of contraception, less than 8% were aware of the full range at their disposal. Nurses must therefore continually update their knowledge of this subject if they are to offer valid and reliable information.

Hormonal contraception

Contraceptive steroids work by preventing ovulation and interfering with the production of Gonadotrophic Releasing Hormone (GnRH) from the hypothalamus. They are taken orally and consist of one of the following:

◇ A fixed-dose combination pill with ethinyloestradiol
◇ A combination of oestrogen and progesterone given daily for 21 days
◇ Progestogen-only pills.

Combined oral contraceptives

The combined oral contraceptives (COC), containing both oestrogen and progesterone, are over 99% effective when taken properly (Andrews 2000), but have side effects of nausea, breast tenderness and fluid retention, which may make their use intolerable for some women. Menstrual bleeding occurs over 3–4 days, and the volume of blood lost is less than would be expected were the pill not being taken.

Several 'pill scares' caused women to transfer to other forms of contraception in 1995, although some stopped using the COC immediately and did not seek an alternative sufficiently quickly to prevent pregnancy, with the consequence that there was a significant rise in abortions during 1996. This occurred across the age range, but especially amongst teenage women.

The scares were mainly related to venous thromboembolism, but in 1999 the Committee on Safety of Medicines (CSM) reversed its advice to women taking third-generation COCs following a lengthy review of the original research. The review indicated that the risk for thromboembolism was much less than had previously been thought.

The relationship between oestrogens and breast cancer has always been debatable. The collaborative group on Hormone Factors in Breast Cancer (1997) found that there was a relative risk of having breast cancer of 1:24 for women using COCs compared with those who did not. This small risk apparently reduced after cessation of COC use and disappeared after a decade of non-use.

Progestogen-only pills

The developments with this contraceptive pill have not been as great as with other varieties, but it is of great value for women who cannot take oestrogen, e.g. breast-feeding mothers and women with hypertension. It needs to be taken at about the same time every day in order to maintain blood progestogen at contraceptive levels. Guillebaud (2000) asserts that the progestogen-only pill is 99% effective when taken according to instructions, and this is supported by Rosevear (2002).

Side effects include mild depression, irritability and fatigue, and higher doses may impair glucose metabolism.

There may be an initial reduction in pregnancy rates when this pill is stopped, but after two years this has resolved and there is no difference in pregnancy incidence. Several studies of nearly 4000 women with cancer of the cervix showed a significantly increased risk of the disease with increased duration of COC use (Colditz *et al* 1994; Schlesselman 1995), the relative risk being between 1.5 and 2.5. However, the COC appears to be protective against endometrial cancer and, the longer it is used the greater the risk reduction. Rosevear (2002) indicates that the protective effect is apparent within 10 years of use and remained for at least 15 years.

Contraindications to COC use

According to Guillebaud (2000), the following are indicators that COCs should not be used:

◇ Cigarette smoking, particularly in women over 35 years (risk of myocardial infarction)
◇ Cardiovascular disease (risk of thromboembolism)
◇ History of malignancy (risk of recurrence)

◇ Hypertension (risk of cardiovascular disease)
◇ Diabetes with retinopathy (risk of increased glucose metabolism impairment)

It is therefore essential that any woman contemplating COC use should be checked for any previous history of the above and further investigated if there is a family history of cardiovascular disease, cervical cancer or diabetes mellitus.

Drug interactions

COCs may be less effective themselves or interfere with the action of several drugs, most notably barbiturates, sulphonamides, cyclophosphamide and rifampicin. There may also be COC failure implications with the use of antibiotics of the penicillin group, some analgesics and phenytoin (Rosevear 2002).

Injectable contraceptives

Injections can be given which bring about contraception for 1, 2 or 3 months. There are several monthly injections, which combine oestrogen and progesterone, but the two- and three-monthly injections are more commonly prescribed.

Medroxyprogesterone acetate (Depo-Provera) is given in 150 mg doses and is effective for 12 weeks. It was granted a licence in 1994 and has been found to be associated with a pregnancy rate of only 0.1% after 1 year. It can cause amenorrhoea in up to 60% of women, with another 30% experiencing metrorrhagia and spotting. Nevertheless, most women will resume normal menstrual cycles within 1 year of discontinuing Depo-Provera (Rosevear 2002).

Norethindrone enanthate (NET-EN or Noristerat) 200 mg is injected at two-monthly intervals initially, and is reported to be as effective as Depo-Provera in preventing pregnancy. After 6 months it can be given at 12-week intervals (World Health Organization 1998). The advantages and disadvantages of its use are similar to those of Depo-Provera.

Hormone Implants

The Family Planning Association (FPA) (1998) reported that, following a five-year study, the progestogen implant Norplant provided over 99% effective contraception. The six small tubes that were implanted subcutaneously in the inner upper arm slowly released levonorgestrel for 60 months. Some women found the tubes uncomfortable and reported difficulty in their removal if contraception became unwanted before the end of the 60 month activity.

Edwards and Moore (1999) found zero failures in over 70,000 cycles from a newer, single rod implant called Implanon, which superseded Norplant in the Autumn of that year. This releases an alternative progestogen – etonogestrel – which has a three-year effective life.

Intrauterine devices (IUDs)

These relatively inexpensive devices generally have a high tolerability by women, and are highly effective in preventing conception. Another benefit is that, following insertion (which may be uncomfortable for some recipients), they are effective for the long term and do not interfere with the spontaneity of sexual intercourse. Once inserted, they can be virtually forgotten, other than the occasional self-check for the attached threads, which can be located in the vagina. Checking for the presence of the threads is essential, as there is a 10% spontaneous expulsion rate (Rosevear 2002).

There are two main types of IUD or coil:

◇ Copper-containing IUDs initiate a foreign body response in the endometrium, which presents a hostile environment to sperm. Contrary to wide belief, the copper containing coils do not affect ovarian function, nor do they act as an abortifacient. Rather, they prevent fertilisation in the vast majority of cases due to spermicidal action.

The FPA (1998) reported IUDs to be over 99% effective, depending on the type used, and recommended the copper-containing IUD post termination of pregnancy for its instant efficacy.

There are adverse effects, including a 10% expulsion rate and up to 1% pregnancy during the first year. Up to 15% of women have the IUD removed due to menorrhagia and severe dysmenorrhoea.

◇ Progestogen-releasing intrauterine system (IUS): this represents a significant improvement in contraception during recent years, and is available as a small, plastic T-shaped structure containing levonorgestrel – the 'Mirena'. It was introduced as a contraceptive in 1995 and the FPA (1998) reported an efficacy of over 99%. The mode of action is to suppress endometrial proliferation, therefore providing a hostile environment for implantation. Additionally, it increases cervical mucus viscosity, causing an effective barrier to sperm penetration. Andrews (2000) asserts that, whilst anovulation can occur, most women using the Mirena will continue to ovulate. It is effective for five years, reduces menorrhagia, dysmenorrhoea and can be inserted at any time of the menstrual cycle. However, unlike the copper IUD, six weeks must elapse post-partum prior to its insertion. It can cause irregular spotting or amenorrhoea, both of which can be of concern to the woman.

In family planning clinics, it is becoming common practice for nurses to be trained to prescribe oral contraceptives and to insert IUDs, thus providing a more comfortable setting, particularly for teenage women, who may be reluctant to discuss sexual issues with a doctor.

It is essential therefore that nurses can advise their clients of the effects and side-effects of all contraceptive methods available in an unemotional and unbiased manner.

There were 40,966 teenage pregnancies in the age range of 15–17 in England and Wales in 2001, rising to 41,868 in 2002 (Teenage Pregnancy Unit 2004), and this increase does little to approach the government's target of reducing the pregnancy rate of under 18s by 50% by the year 2010. The Unit did recognise that the 10 year strategy, including disseminating information about individually suited contraception, needs to be sustained over a long period in order to effect behavioural and social change. Nurses are therefore in an ideal position to break down communication barriers in schools and family planning clinics, doctor's surgeries and 'walk-in' centres.

Emergency contraception

The probability of pregnancy following a single act of sexual intercourse during the four days preceding ovulation is 20%, but this is increased to 30% on the day of ovulation. At other times of the cycle it is usually less than 10%.

If unprotected sexual intercourse has occurred on day 13 or 14 of a 28-day cycle, emergency post-coital contraception should be available to females requesting it.

Andrews (2000) comments upon the numerous campaigns during the 1990s aimed at raising public awareness of the availability of emergency contraception and outlines the two main traditional methods:

◇ The Yuzpe method was, until recently the most commonly used regimen, and prevented 75% of pregnancies that would have otherwise resulted. The woman is given 100 micrograms (µg) of ethinyloestradiol + 500 µg levonorgestrel, with the regime repeated 12 hours later. The therapy needs to be commenced within 72 hours of unprotected sexual intercourse. Some GPs recommend prescribing an extra two tablets in case the patient vomited within 3 hours of ingestion of the originals.

◇ IUD insertion within 5 days of unprotected intercourse or within 5 days of the estimated time of ovulation.

With both types, efficacy decreases with increasing time since unprotected sexual intercourse.

In 1998 the Task Force on Postovulatory Methods of Fertility Regulation published results of a comparative trial which indicated that Levonorgestrel 0.75 mg, repeated 12 hours later (Postinor 2) was better tolerated than the Yuzpe regime and was more effective. Effectiveness, however, as with other emergency contraception programmes, is reduced as the time between intercourse and commencement of therapy increases. It was licensed for emergency contraception in the UK in 2000, and is now more widely followed than the two traditional methods.

The Task Force on Postovulatory Methods of Fertility Regulation (1999) concluded that, as an alternative emergency contraceptive, mifepristone (RU486) 600 mg given within 72 hours of unprotected sexual intercourse has been associated with zero pregnancies and is therefore a useful adjunct to therapeutic choices.

The dose of 600 mg significantly delays the next menstrual period, which may be anxiety-provoking for the woman who is not intent on a pregnancy. Mifepristone 10 mg is said to be equally effective in preventing pregnancy, but does not delay the onset of the next menstrual period, and therefore is likely to be more acceptable to women requiring this type of contraception. There needs to be more research in this area to compare mifepristone and levonorgestrel for pros and cons.

Both therapies cause less nausea and vomiting than the Yuzpe regime, thereby increasing their acceptability over the latter.

Because of the nature of emergency contraception, some level of sexual health promotion is essential in that:

◇ The woman needs to have knowledge and control of her own fertility and sexual responses.
◇ She needs to understand how (if used), a particular contraceptive method has failed and how to prevent this situation recurring.
◇ She should understand the risk of sexually transmitted diseases from unprotected casual coitus, particularly chlamydia, which may be asymptomatic but can, at a later stage, cause ectopic pregnancy and infertility (Social Exclusion Unit 1999).

As nurses are now more involved in health promotion as well as sickness services, their role in this particular situation is paramount.

Barrier methods of contraception

Male

The male condom is probably one of the oldest barrier methods of contraception, some early prototypes being thought to have been made from animal hide and with a single condom designed for use by the man throughout his adult sexual life.

Modern condoms are manufactured from vulcanised latex rubber or polyurethane and are designed for single use only. The condom is, to date, the only reliable method of male contraception, apart from vasectomy, with a reported 98% effectiveness rating when appropriately used (FPA 1998).

In addition, the latex rubber condom is protective against gonorrhoea, HIV, trichomonas vaginitis, hepatitis B, syphilis, herpes simplex and chlamydia in the female, provided that chemical interactions used during sexual intercourse do not interfere with the latex durability. Water-based lubricants, glycerol and silicones are safe to use with this type of condom.

In 1997, due to increasing reports of latex allergies, a new polyurethane condom became available which is thinner but stronger than latex and is unharmed by oil-based lubricants/spermicides. It is transparent and odourless, and for these reasons may become more widely acceptable than the latex variety, thereby assisting the fight against sexually transmitted diseases.

Andrews (2000) reports that there are several 'fumble-free' variations that prevent male condoms from being applied inside out, giving the 'Topaz' condom as an example.

Female

The first female condom, 'Femidom', became available in the UK in 1992 and is reported to have a 95% success rate, when correctly adopted (FPA 1998). It too, offers protection against HIV and other sexually transmitted diseases, and is made of polyurethane material with similar qualities to the male polyurethane condom. Bounds *et al* (1992) noted that the Femidom rarely tears and that men report less loss of sensitivity than with the male condom; it is as easily obtained but may interfere with the spontaneity of sexual intercourse due to its 'rustling' sound when used.

Caps and diaphragms achieve an approximate success rate of 94% according to the FPA (1998) when correctly used, but Bounds *et al* (1995) recommend the additional use of spermicide in order to maintain this rate. They may be inserted prior to intercourse and are designed to fit snugly over the cervix, therefore effectively denying sperm access to the cervical os. Women do need to practice inserting these devices as they are not available in 'one size fits all', which may be one reason for the fact that their use is not widespread.

Guillebaud (1993) asserts that these also offer protection from pelvic infection and cervical cell dysplasia, but not from HIV infection and similar sexually transmitted organisms.

Sterilisation

Male

Vasectomy or male sterilisation involves surgical severing or diathermy of bilateral vasa deferentia. The vas deferens is a tube that transports sperm, manufactured in the seminal vesicles, to the exit point of the penile shaft, having conjoined with the urethra just below the bladder. Both the prostate gland and seminal vesicles contribute to the process of ejaculation and transportation of seminal fluid and sperms to the cervix for fertilisation to occur.

Bilateral vasectomy provides a quick, easy and effective method of contraception which can be performed under local anaesthetic – the most preferred choice, according to Black and Francome (2002) – or a general anaesthetic.

Gormley (2003) quotes a figure of 99.9% efficacy and argues that bilateral vasectomy has no effect on sexual functioning, but there may be overriding psychological problems for some men who would therefore reject the offer of permanent sterility.

The surgical procedure usually takes no longer than 15 minutes and is safer and simpler than female sterilisation procedures. However, given that its safety, simplicity and effectiveness are highly rated, the permanency of the surgical technique must be conveyed to the man contemplating sterilisation. He must understand, when agreeing to the procedure, that its effect is not immediate – two negative semen analyses, three months after the vasectomy, taken at about a four-week interval will be required to establish sterility. Even so, this is not a guaranteed outcome, as in some cases sperm clearance can take longer.

During surgery, a small incision or puncture is made on each side of the scrotum, and the vasa are pulled through the entry point. The vasa may then be either cut, and a small portion removed and the cut ends ligated, or sealed by electrocauterisation (Black and Francome 2002). As the wound is tiny, it may simply be covered by a small gauze dressing or butterfly tape sutures if needed.

The nursing role may include involvement in counselling prior to the procedure, when the possibility of failure of the surgical intervention must be addressed. Belfield (1999) asserts that this has approximately a 1:2000 lifetime rate and that reversing the procedure is difficult and frequently unsuccessful.

Post-operative care is usually carried out by the nurse, who will check for haematoma development and bleeding prior to discharge. The nurse will also provide the patient with verbal and written instructions for further self-care to enable an uncomplicated recovery.

Semen analysis sampling details will be given as well as advice regarding the avoidance of heavy lifting for 1 to 2 weeks post surgery. It is important to stress the need to continue with additional contraception until the semen samples have proven negative; however, sexual activity may resume when the patient is comfortable and pain-free.

Advice from the nurse about possible complications should be offered. These include infections and haematomae, both of which are relatively easily resolved. Sperm granuloma – leaking of sperms into the tissue between the severed vasa deferentia – may cause pain and swelling that might require surgical removal (Everett 2001).

Whilst some vasectomised men, or those considering this contraceptive method, might be concerned about the surgical intervention and a link with prostatic cancer, De Antoni (1997) studied more than 95,000 men involved in prostate cancer screening, with results that indicated no higher risk in vasectomised males, compared with the non-vasectomised participants.

Dawe and Meltzer (2001) reported that about 45% of couples aged over 40 in the UK use sterilisation as a contraceptive technique, which offers the freedom of sexual intercourse without the possibility of an unwanted pregnancy and the added benefit of total spontaneity.

The fact that some men may grieve about their perceived 'loss of masculinity' and possible sexual dysfunction/impotence should be addressed by effective pre- and post-operative discussion.

Gormley (2003) states that:

> There are no standardised guidelines for vasectomy reversal. The procedure may be available on the NHS if the man has been on the waiting list for 18 months.

She states that the success rates of reversal vary widely and relate to several factors, including when the vasectomy was undertaken, the specific type of surgery, presence of any antibodies and the surgical skills of the operator. It must be accepted that the possibility of any future pregnancy resulting from a reversed vasectomy is also influenced by the woman's fertility potential.

Female

In women, sterilisation involves obstructing the fallopian tubes, thereby preventing the ovum (released cyclically from the ovary) and the sperm (ascending the female reproductive tract following ejaculation) from meeting, and fertilisation ensuing.

As with vasectomy in the male, this procedure should be considered to be permanent and irreversible; thus full and appropriate discussion with health professionals must be available, and should include the possibility of surgical failure. Equally, many surgeons wish to ensure the agreement of opposite sex partners, but that person's consent is not legally required for the surgery to proceed.

The most common method of female sterilisation in the UK is via a laparoscopic approach through the abdominal wall, locating and tying each fallopian tube in two places, and then removing a small section of the tube between the ligatures. The same effect may be achieved by sealing the tubes bilaterally using cautery/diathermy, or by application of 'clothes peg' type Filshie clips or Falope rings.

The procedure may be undertaken as an inpatient or an outpatient, using general or local anaesthetic, and the woman is usually able to return home after a maximum of 24 hours. Alternative contraception methods should be employed until she has experienced her first port-operative menstrual period.

The effectiveness of female sterilisation is reputed to be a lifetime failure of 1 in 200 (Belfield 1999). However, earlier research from Peterson *et al* (1996) indicated that recanalisation of the fallopian tubes following surgical obstruction may be greater than had previously been reported. It may fail several years post-surgery and the failure rate is affected by the surgeon's approach and surgical ability in securing the appropriate result.

Nurses will be involved in post-operative care and possibly with pre-operative discussion, particularly where nurse-led, pre-admission clinics are in operation. It is important that such discussions should be delayed if predisposing partnership/marital problems prevail or if the woman has recently suffered a spontaneous or planned termination of pregnancy, as these events may have an influence over the decision that might subsequently be regretted.

Additionally, when either male or female sterilisation is being planned, any psychiatric illness should be considered as misinterpretation of the effects of surgery could have implications for future mental health stability.

There are few side-effects following female sterilisation – ovulation and menstruation continue as previously – but should an unwanted pregnancy occur, the risk of an ectopic pregnancy is about 33% (Peterson *et al* 1996). Sexual intercourse may be resumed when the woman feels comfortable, and for many enjoyment is improved due to the removed fear of an unwanted pregnancy.

Because the diversity of practice in the UK, the RCOG (1999) produced national guidelines in order to standardise counselling, training and surgical practice.

Conclusion

Rapid changes in contraception, the rise in sexually transmitted diseases and large numbers of teenage pregnancies in the UK have all contributed to increased knowledge of male and female fertility during the last decade. It is therefore essential that all nurses keep up to date with issues surrounding conception, contraception, fertility and infertility, and be willing to discuss these very personal and intimate issues with patients, within an atmosphere of compassion and discretion.

References

Abbott, L (2004) Ectopic pregnancy: symptoms, diagnosis and management. *Nursing Times* **100**(6) 32–33

Action on Smoking and Health (2001) *Smoking and Health Inequalities.* ASH, NHS Health Development Agency, London

Ahmed, M S, Cemerikic, B and Agbas A (1992) Properties of functions of the human placental opioid system: a review. *Life Sciences* **50** 83–97

Allanach, V (2003) in Radcliffe, M (2003) Fertile ground. *Nursing Times* **99**(1) 42–43

Andrews, G (2000) Contraception: what has changed over the past decade? *Nursing Times*9(6) 326–332

Ankum, W M (2000) Diagnosing suspected ectopic pregnancies. *British Journal of Medicine* **321** 1235–1236

Balen, A H (1997) Anovulatory fertility and ovulation induction. Policy and Practice Subcommittee of the British Fertility Society. *Human Reproduction* **12** (Supplement II) 83–87

Belker, A M, Thomas, A J, Fuchs, E F and Konnak, J (1991) Results of 1469 microsurgical vasectomy reversals by the Vasovasectomy Study Group. *Journal of Urology* **145** 505–511

Belfield, T (1999) *Contraceptive Handbook.* Family Planning Association, London

Ben-Jonathan, N, Laudon, M and Garris, P A (1991) Novel aspects of posterior pituitary function: regulation of prolactin secretion. *Frontiers in Neuroendocrinology* **12** 231–277

Black, T and Francome, C (2002) The evolution of the Marie Stopes electrocautery, no-scalpel vasectomy procedure. *Journal of Family Planning and Reproductive Health Care* **28**(3) 137–138

Bounds, W, Guillebaud, J J and Newman, G (1992) Female condom (Femidom): a clinical study of its use, effectiveness and patient acceptability. *British Journal of Family Planning* **18**(2) 36–41

Bounds, W, Guillebaud, J J and Dominik R (1995) The diaphragm with and without spermicide: a randomised comparative efficacy trial. *Journal of Reproductive Medicine* **40**(11) 764–774

Brown, J (1999) The effect of clinician communication skills on client satisfaction: a randomised controlled trial. *Annals of International Medicine* **131**(11) 822–829

Burns, C (2003) Sperm bank plea for new donors. *Leicester Mercury*, 19 Sept, p. 8

Chubb, E and Knight, J (1996) *Fertility.* David & Charles, Newton Abbott

Clancy, J and McVicar, A (2002) *Physiology and Anatomy.* Arnold, London

Colditz, G A (1994) Oral contraceptive use and mortality during 12 years follow-up: the Nurses' Health Study. *Internal Medicine* **120** 821–825

Collaborative Group on Hormone Factors in Breast Cancer (1997) Collaborative re-analysis of data from 51 epidemiological studies of 51,705 women with breast cancer and 108,411 women without breast cancer. *Lancet* **350** 1047–1059

Collins, J A, Burrows, E A and Willan, A R (1995) The prognosis for live birth among untreated infertile couples. *Fertility and Sterility* **64** 22–28

Dawe, F and Meltzer, H (2001) *Contraception and Sexual Health.* Office for National Statistics, London

De Antoni, E R (1997) A cross-sectional study of vasectomy, time since vasectomy and prostate cancer. *Prostatic Cancer and Prostatic Disease* **1** 73–78

Department of Health (1992) *The Health of The Nation.* DoH, London

Department of Health (1999) *Saving Lives, Our Healthier Nation*. DoH, London

Ectopic Pregnancy Trust (2004) `http://www.ectopic.org.uk/`

Edwards, J E and Moore A (1999) Implanon: a review of clinical studies. *British Journal of Family Planning* **24** 3–16

Everett, S (2001) Contraception. In Andrews, G (ed) *Women's Sexual Health*. Ballière Tindall, London

Family Planning Association (1998) *Your Guide to Contraception*. FPA, London

Fischel, S, Green, S and Bishop, M (1995) Pregnancy after intracytoplasmic injection of spermatid. *Lancet* **345** 1641–1642

Fischel, S, Dowell, K, Timson, J and Green S (1993) Micro-assisted fertilisation with human gametes. *Human Reproduction* **8** 1780–1784

Fleming, L (2003) Moments of such supreme happiness. *Nursing Times* **99**(1) 43

Garrow, J (1991) Treating obesity. *British Medical Journal* **302** 804–809

Gilbert, G L (ed) (1993) Infectious diseases: challenges for the 1990s. In: Ballières Clinical Obstetrics and Gynaecology. *International Practice and Research* **17**(1) 159–193

Gillick v West Norfolk and Wisbech AHA and the DHSS (1985) 3 All ER 402

Gormley, M (2003) Ensuring that having a vasectomy is an informed decision. *Nursing Times* **99**(46) 28–30

Greenhall, E and Vessey, M (1990) The prevalence of subfertility: a review of current confusion and a report of two new studies. *Fertility and Sterility* **54** 978–983

Guillebaud, J J (1993) *Contraception: Four Questions Answered*. Churchill Livingstone, Edinburgh

Guillebaud, J J (2000) *Contraception Today*, 4th edn. Martin Dunitz, London

Health Education Authority (1996) *Think About Drink, There's More to Drink than You Think*. HEA, London

Herman, J (1997) *Trauma and Recovery*. HarperCollins, New York

Hughes, E G and Brennan, B G (1996) Does cigarette smoking impair natural or assisted fecundity? *Fertility and Sterility* **66** 679–689

Human Fertilisation and Embryology Authority (1994) *Third Annual Report*. HFEA, London

Human Fertilisation and Embryology Authority (1995) *The Patient Guide to DI and IVF Clinics*. HFEA, London

Human Fertilisation and Embryology Authority (2003) `http://www.hfea.gov.uk/`

Human Fertilisation and Embryology Authority (2004) *HFEA Supports Human Cloning in the UK*. http://www.globalchange.com/

Jain, K (1988) Comparison of transvaginal and transabdominal sonography in the detection of an early pregnancy and its complications. *American Journal of Radiology* **151** 1139–43

Mack, S and Tucker, J (1996) *Fertility Counselling*. Baillière Tindall, London

Mieusset, R and Bujan, L (1995) Testicular heating and its possible contribution to male infertility: a review. *International Journal of Andrology* **18** 169–184

Murdoch, A (2003) Free IVF Plan Welcomed. *Daily Telegraph*, 26 Aug, p. 9

National Institute for Clinical Excellence (2003) http://www.nice.org.uk/

National Statistics (2003) *Social Trends*. HMSO, London

Nursing and Midwifery Council (2002a) *Guidelines for Professional Practice*. NMC, London

Nursing and Midwifery Council (2002b) *Code of Professional Conduct*. NMC, London

Payne, L (2003) Should aborted foetus cells aid infertile adults? *Nursing Times* **99**(39) 19

Peterson, P, Xia, Z and Hughes, J M (1996) The risk of pregnancy after tubal sterilisation: findings from the US Collaborative Review of Sterilisation. *American Journal of Obstetrics and Gynaecology* **174**(4) 1161–1170

Pollard, I (1994) *A Guide to Reproduction*. Cambridge University Press, Cambridge

Radcliffe, M (2003) Fertile ground. *Nursing Times* **99**(1) 43

Reid, J (2004) Free IVF treatment for women under 40. *Daily Telegraph*, 24 Feb, p. 5

Rosevear, S (2002) *Handbook of Gynaecological Management*. Blackwell Science, Oxford

Rossing, M A, Daling, J R, Weiss, N S, Moore, D E and Self, S G (1994) Ovarian tumours in a cohort of infertile women. *New England Journal of Medicine* **331**, 771–776

Royal College of Obstetricians and Gynaecologists (1998) *Management Of Infertile Couples: Evidence-based Clinical Guidelines No 2*. RCOG, London

Royal College of Obstetricians and Gynaecologists (1999) *Male and Female Sterilisation: Evidence-Based Guidelines No 5*. RCOG, London

Royal College of Obstetricians and Gynaecologists (2002) *Clinical Guidelines for Tubal Pregnancies*. RCOG, London

Schlesselman, J J (1995) Net effect of oral contraceptive use on the risk of cancer in women in the United States. *Obstetrics and Gynaecology* **85** 793–891

Sizoo, L (2002) *Small Sparks of Life*. Groningen, Netherlands, Gopher Publishers

Social Exclusion Unit (1999) *Teenage Pregnancy*. SEU, London

Stabile, L (1996) *Ectopic Pregnancy; Diagnosis and Management*. Cambridge University Press, Cambridge

Steptoe, P C and Edwards, R G (1978) Birth after the reimplantation of a human embryo (letter). *The Lancet* **ii** (8085) 366

Task Force on Postovulatory Methods of Fertility Regulation (1998) Randomised controlled trial of levonorgestrel versus the Yuzpe regimen of combined oral contraceptives for emergency contraception. *Lancet* **352** 428–433

Task Force on Postovulatory Methods of Fertility Regulation (1999) Comparison of 3 single doses of mifepristone as emergency contraception: a randomised trial. *Lancet* **353** 697–702

Tay J (2000) Ectopic pregnancy. *British Journal of Medicine* **320** 916–919

Te Velde, E R, Eijkemans, R and Habbema, H D (2000) Variations in couple fecundity and time to pregnancy, an essential concept in human reproduction. *The Lancet* **355** 1928–1929

Teenage Pregnancy Unit (2004) UK pregnancy rate increases. *Nursing Times* **100**(11) 7

Whyte, D and Donaldson, J (1999) All in the family. *Nursing Times* **95**(32) 48

Whittaker, N (2004) *Disorders and Interventions*. Palgrave, Basingstoke

Wilkie, J C (2003) I'm pro life and oppose embryonic stem cell research. http://www.lifeissues.org/cloningstemcell/

Winston, R (1994) *Infertility*. Optima, London

Womack, S (2003) Put family on hold. *Daily Telegraph*, 14 Nov, p. 5

World Health Organization (1998) *WHO Scientific Group on Cardiovascular Disease: Steroid Hormone Contraception*. Report of a WHO Scientific Group, WHO, Geneva

Yao, M and Tulandi, T (1997) Current status of surgical and non-surgical management of ectopic pregnancy. *Fertility and Sterility* **67** 421–433

Useful addresses and web sites

CHILD (The National Infertility Support Network)

Charter House

43 St Leonards Road, Bexhill on Sea, East Sussex TN40 1JA

01424 732361

ISSUE (The National Fertility Association)
509 Aldridge Road, Great Barr, Birmingham B44 8NA
0121 344 4414

HFEA
Paxton House, 30 Artillery Road, London E1 7LS
0207 3775077
http://www.hfea.gov.uk/

National Gamete Donation Trust
http://www.ngdt.co.uk/
0161 276 6000

Donor Conception Network
http://www.dcnetwork.org/
020 8245 4369

The Assisted Conception Unit
University College Hospital, London
http://www.conception-acu.com/

COTS
http://www.surrogacy.org.uk/

Ectopic Pregnancy Trust
c/o Maternity Unit, Hillingdon Hospital, Red Heath Rd, Uxbridge, Middlesex UB8 3NN
01895 238025
http://www.ectopic.org.uk/

Family Planning Information Service
27–35 Mortimer Street, London W1N 7RJ

CHAPTER 2

Abortion

Introduction

This chapter addresses the contentious issue of abortion, both planned and spontaneous. It discusses past, present and potential future incidences and trends, offering possible predisposing factors to peaks and troughs that have occurred, and which may be repeated in future.

Legal issues are included. Both medical and surgical management of the abortion process are presented and the role of nurses in relation to both will be discussed.

Definition and statistics

Abortion is the generic name given to termination of pregnancy which occurs either accidentally (spontaneous abortion, or miscarriage) or as a planned medical/surgical discontinuation of the pregnancy.

Planned abortion rates vary according to the age of women, with those under 16 years and those over 30 years having lower rates than all other age groups. In 2001 the rate for under 16s was 3.7 per 1000 pregnancies, and for pregnant women over 35 years the rate was 6.4 per 1000 pregnancies (National Statistics 2003).

The Abortion Act, which became law in 1967, was passed in anticipation of Furedi (1996):

◇ reducing morbidity and mortality arising from so-called 'back street' abortions – those performed illegally and usually by medically unqualified persons, and

◇ the improved availability and efficacy of contraceptive methods and therefore, the expectation that the numbers of women seeking abortion would decline

However, this anticipated decline in abortion rates has not materialised. In fact, the numbers have increased dramatically, particularly for women in the age group 16–24 years. In 2001, National Statistics (2003) reported that 26.1 per 1000 pregnant women in the 16–19 years age range aborted their pregnancies, as opposed to 6.1 per 1000 in 1969, rising from 7 per 1000 pregnancies aborted in that year, to 30.6 per 1000 in 2001.

In 1997, the vast majority of terminations – almost 90% – were carried out before 13 weeks gestation (Mahoney 1997), and in 1998 almost half of abortions took place before 9 weeks, compared with about 34% in 1986. Almost three-quarters of these were undertaken by the National Health Service (NHS), compared with 50% in the years 1986–1991.

Several factors influence the above figures, many of which could not have been foreseen in 1967 when the Abortion Act was passed; these factors include contraceptive pill 'scares'. In 1995–96 a temporary increase in abortion rates was recorded following a report by the Commission on Safety of Medicines warning of links with the drugs and thromboembolic disease.

Unfortunately, the predicted decline to the pre-1995 abortion rate did not happen, which may have been due to continued warnings linking the 'pill' to thrombosis generally, and to deep vein thrombosis connected to the increase in long-haul air flights (National Statistics 2003).

Prior to the 1967 Abortion Act, termination of pregnancy could be carried out, but only to preserve the mother's life. The Act itself extended the grounds for abortion to be carried out legally in this country, but these are controlled and statistics carefully monitored.

In the 1967 Act (which drew from the Infant Life Preservation Act 1929 and the Offences Against The Person Act 1861) termination of pregnancy could be legally undertaken up to 28 weeks gestation, provided that two medically qualified practitioners agreed upon one of the four grounds set out in the Act under section 1 (1), these being:

◇ The risk of continuing the pregnancy would compromise the life of the pregnant woman
◇ The continuance of the pregnancy would involve serious risk to the mental health of the woman
◇ The continuation of the pregnancy would seriously affect the physical or mental health of any existing children of the family of the pregnant woman
◇ There would be a substantial risk of the child being born seriously handicapped

The criteria for abortion would be based upon a discussion between the pregnant woman and, usually, her general practitioner and the doctor performing the termination. Several factors would be considered, including the pregnant woman's current social situation, environmental influences such as housing, and financial support for children for whom she is taking responsibility.

Numerous parliamentary debates arose as a result of pressure groups lobbying Members of Parliament to either tighten, relax or abolish the 1967 Act, which culminated in an amendment to it by section 37 of the Human Fertilisation and Embryology Act 1990, which became operational in 1992.

It had been recognised that medical diagnostic and treatment skills had advanced considerably during the period between the 1967 Abortion Act and the health situation of 1990, whereby a foetus which might have been aborted at 28 weeks in 1967 and not survived could have a reasonable chance of survival given appropriate medical attention by the year 1990.

Factors including improved sex and health education of teenagers (Kiddy 2002), greater access to genetics clinics (where tests can be undertaken to help determine the possibilities of passing on undesirable inherited diseases such as Huntington's chorea), and hugely advanced predictive technology, meant that changes to the 1967 Abortion Act needed to be made.

Those changes were within the 'Certificate of Opinion' which has to be agreed by the two medical practitioners who have attended the pregnant woman under section 1 (1) of the Act. The amendments relate to the individual pregnant woman's situation, and have to be identified by both medical practitioners as either:

◇ the continuance of the pregnancy would involve risk to the life of the pregnant woman, greater than if the pregnancy were terminated;

◇ the termination is necessary to prevent grave permanent injury to the physical or mental health of the pregnant woman;

◇ the pregnancy has NOT exceeded its 24th week and that the continuance of the pregnancy would involve risk, greater than if the pregnancy were terminated, of injury to the physical or mental health of the pregnant woman;

◇ the pregnancy has NOT exceeded its 24th week and that the continuance of the pregnancy would involve risk, greater than if the pregnancy were terminated, of injury to the physical or mental health of any existing child(ren) of the family of the pregnant woman;

◇ there is substantial risk that if the child were born it would suffer from such physical or mental abnormalities as to be seriously handicapped.

The amendment therefore gives the upper time limit of 24 weeks for termination of pregnancy, with the exception of some extreme circumstances, but does not alter the principles of the 1967 Act, nor deny access to women who would previously have been able to request a legal termination of pregnancy.

According to Belfield (1999), although abortion has always been, and continues to be, a controversial issue of mental health:

The extent to which legislation follows or influences public opinion, is debatable.

Whilst various opinion polls have indicated that there is a strong public view that abortion should be available 'on request', the prevailing situation is that there is *no* legal requirement for health authorities to provide an abortion service. Hence there is considerable variation between services available across localities.

Abortion is available privately, but clinics offering this provision have to be registered as approved by the Department of Health and inspected regularly to ensure that standards are maintained.

Counselling of the pregnant woman and partner (if appropriate) should always be available, but given the necessity for a speedy decision in order to limit physical and psychological complications, a number of people may not wish to avail themselves of this service, or may be resolute before the service is offered.

Termination of pregnancy (TOP)

The safest time for TOP is within the first trimester and can be carried out either medically or surgically.

◇ *Medical*
   Since 1995 the licence for mifepristone use in abortion has been approved for gestations up to 20 weeks (Furedi 1996) and Spitz *et al* (1998) indicated a success rate of nearly 90% during the first trimester when oral mifepristone, combined with the prostaglandin misoprostol inserted vaginally, resulted in termination usually within 8 hours.
◇ *Surgical*
   – Dilatation and curettage (D&C) is carried out less frequently than other methods, but can be used up to 12 weeks gestation in young women up to 18 years. Cervical softening via one of

the prostaglandin preparations is usual prior to the D&C, which is carried out with the patient lightly anaesthetised (Belfield 1999).

– Suction/vacuum aspiration is more commonly undertaken than D&C and the operation is carried out usually under local or light general anaesthetic. The cervix is dilated and the uterine contents evacuated via a small bore plastic tube.

Both medical and surgical terminations may be performed in an NHS hospital or place approved by the Secretary of State for Health or by the Secretary of State for Scotland.

Generally, TOP before 12 weeks gestation is safe and easy to accomplish, but as with all medical/surgical procedures, there are possible complications – in this case, a very low mortality rate of less than 1 in 1,000,000 with surgically induced terminations, and a failure of termination of 3 in 1000 women. Incomplete termination occurs in about 2 in 100, but with medical TOP about a quarter of women suffer from nausea and vomiting, and a small percentage from diarrhoea. Very few women suffer from significant blood loss, with only 1 in 2000 requiring replacement therapy (Rosevear 2002).

The nurse's role in the above is to treat the patient with respect (since there may be guilt feelings being held by the woman seeking TOP, who may interpret a nurse's unconscious body language in a negative way) and to welcome her to the ward or clinic. It is obvious that those women who are admitted to a gynaecological ward in hospital should not be placed in an area where women who are undergoing investigations or treatment for infertility are also situated – nurses must be sensitive to the feelings of both. Indeed, if nurses cannot themselves accept this dichotomy, then they should question their ability to care effectively, in a non-judgemental manner, for women with either need.

The nurse should be positive in approach, knowledgeable about the procedure that the woman is about to undergo and be able to answer questions and allay any fears regarding the termination of pregnancy.

She must also be conversant with methods of contraception about which the patient may request information.

Preparation of the woman for treatment must be efficient but sensitive, with consideration towards privacy for the patient and any friend or partner she has accompanying her. Confidentiality may be a concern for the woman and the nurse must ensure that this is fully maintained (NMC 2002) and clear informed consent established. Nurses sometimes view the 'consent to medical/surgical treatment' as solely the medical role, but given that nurses should offer 'holistic' care, they must ensure that the patient has total understanding of the procedure that she is about to undergo, and of the possible (but uncommon) complications.

Late abortions

Medical

Pregnancies of over 13 weeks, and particularly those between 15 and 20 weeks usually require prostaglandin termination, as foetal parts are more difficult to evacuate by suction evacuation. Vaginal prostaglandins are given in combination with mifepristone or misoprostol and a 'mini labour' is induced.

Women undergoing this procedure must be given full information as to the reasons for its use in preference to surgery, since some might feel that they are being 'punished' (Spitz *et al* 1998) by health professionals for their decision to end the pregnancy. The uterine contractions induced by the prostaglandins cause cervical dilatation and evacuation of the products of conception.

It is usual to follow the medical termination with a gentle suction curettage under light anaesthetic to ensure complete emptying of the uterus. As the medical procedure can cause cervical tearing, an assessment for this complication must be made at the time of surgical intervention and corrected to avoid future cervical incompetence and loss of prospective wanted pregnancy.

Some women also suffer from troublesome side-effects such as diarrhoea and vomiting, particularly when prostaglandins are administered intravenously. A more effective delivery of the drugs is via a catheter inserted through the cervix to lie between the uterine wall and amniotic membrane, and Chamberlain (1995) claims that this method is generally more effective and results in less nausea and vomiting.

Nurses need to use their communication, observational and practical skills during this time to ensure maximum comfort for women who may become very distressed from side-effects.

Surgical

The later that surgical terminations are carried out, the more likely complications are to arise. However, legal terminations can be performed up to the 24th week of pregnancy, and those between 20–24 weeks are usually conducted via an abdominal hysterotomy. This may be described as a 'mini Caesarean Section' which is performed under general anaesthetic, and is usually necessary because abnormalities of foetal development have been undetected until late in the pregnancy. This may have a psychologically devastating effect upon the prospective parents.

The operation consists of a low abdominal incision and the uterine wall is incised following an intravenous injection of ergometrine. Uterine contents are removed and the uterus and abdomen are sutured in the normal post-surgical manner.

During hysterotomy, should the woman so desire, tubal ligation to ensure future sterility may be undertaken, but it is essential for health care practitioners to understand that a woman who has come to such a decision at that stage of pregnancy may be so distraught that rationality does not come easily.

Generally, therapeutic TOP is safe when carried out by the medical/surgical procedures already described. There are risks with both legal termination of pregnancy and spontaneous abortion, and deaths do still occur.

The cause of such mortality is usually overwhelming infection. Criminal abortions are still enacted, but in very small numbers following the 1967 Abortion Act, which legalised the procedure. The fact that some women do still feel the need to approach unqualified people to perform such an act, or to try and induce TOP themselves, reignites the question of whether abortion should be available 'on request'.

Spontaneous abortion

This term relates to the unintended loss of a pregnancy before the 24th week and is synonymous with the word miscarriage. The latter is probably a better term to use than 'abortion' to women who have experienced or who are experiencing this phenomenon, as abortion may still carry a notion of stigma for some.

The frequency of spontaneous abortion is difficult to establish since many probably occur very early and the woman may not have realised that she was pregnant, and believe that she has merely had an unusually heavy period. Sometimes failure of implantation of the fertilised egg means that the woman does not miss a period, but Chamberlain (1995) estimates that 10–15% of all confirmed conceptions will spontaneously abort. He also calculates that 25% of women will have experienced loss of an early pregnancy during their reproductive life.

Although the most common time for spontaneous abortion is 8–12 weeks, if a normal ultrasound scan is recorded at 10 weeks such an outcome becomes less likely.

Whilst the cause of spontaneous abortion is unclear, there are several predisposing factors which may lie with either the foetus or mother, including:

◇ Hormonal – some women may not produce sufficient progesterone to allow adequate decidual growth prior to placental development. This leads to improper implantation and loss of the pregnancy.

◇ Trauma – severe injury to the uterus, including surgical intervention, may cause detachment of the early placenta and an inevitable outcome.

◇ Infections – rubella, chlamydia, listeriosis and any organism that causes acute pyrexia have all been linked to early spontaneous abortion, although some may cause intra-uterine death at a later stage in the pregnancy.

◇ Anaemia and malnutrition – if the woman has insufficient reserves of basic nutrients, this may affect the viability of the growing foetus and lead to its loss.

◇ Noxious substances – tobacco smoke (ASH 2001), alcohol, heavy metal poisoning (lead) and some drugs such as cytotoxics, class 'A' drugs (Naidoo and Wills 2000) and quinine have all been implicated in early spontaneous abortion (Chamberlain 1995).

◇ Immunological abnormalities – it is thought that some women fail to produce the antibodies that normally prevent rejection of the 'foreign body' (foetus), causing it to be expelled from the uterus.

◇ Embryo defects – chromosomal abnormalities such as trisomy 23 or XO and XXO aberrations account for around 70% of spontaneous abortions. Fortunately most are single events that have little effect on future pregnancies (Rosevear 2002). However where two or more spontaneous abortions do occur, genetic/chromosomal investigations should be carried out.

Classification of spontaneous abortions

Abortions are classified into several types.

Threatened abortion

This is characterised by sudden, painless, light vaginal bleeding which may increase in quantity. The bleeding is due to slight detachment of the placenta and blood loss into the choriodecidual space, but the cervix is usually closed and the uterus of the appropriate gestational size. Many women will go on to deliver successfully at full term (Chamberlain 1995) and there is little evidence to suggest that any medical intervention makes a positive difference to this situation. However, if the woman develops painful contractions accompanied by heavier vaginal bleeding, the cervix may have begun to dilate, with the likelihood of an inevitable abortion.

It is important to establish the viability of the pregnancy via ultrasound imaging as soon as possible. The presence of foetal cardiac movements is an encouraging sign, since this is usually evident using the scanning technique at 7 weeks of pregnancy. The scan will also detect a twin pregnancy and in some cases one twin may be lost but the second remain viable. It will also identify an ectopic pregnancy and an empty gestational sac, both of which mean loss of the foetus.

Nursing care and communication in an empathetic manner is important at this distressing time and, whilst encouragement is helpful where bleeding is slight or stops, false hope should not be pursued.

Inevitable abortion

If the cervix begins to dilate when an abortion is 'threatened', the loss of the conception becomes inevitable. If this occurs before the end of the first trimester, the uterine contractions are usually sufficient to completely empty the uterine cavity. If the problem arises in the subsequent trimester, the foetus is delivered but placental remnants may be retained which can cause severe complications for the woman.

Nursing interventions include preparation of the patient for surgical removal of placental remains and careful monitoring post-operatively for bleeding, shock and sepsis. Intravenous plasma expanding fluids/blood may be needed and the nurse must ensure that these are safely administered. The patient is usually given intramuscular syntometrine once the uterine evacuation procedure is completed, which assists with controlling the blood loss, but the nurse must be vigilant at this critical time. Occasionally prolonged bleeding following surgical intervention may be unassociated with the abortion and may be due to an innocent polyp or, more sinisterly, a malignancy of the cervix.

Complete abortion

All of the products of conception have been completely evacuated, bleeding reduces and the woman is pain-free. An ultrasound scan will confirm an empty uterus and a closed cervix. This is likely to be a sad time for the woman and partner and the nurse must be sensitive to their feelings. She must also warn the woman to report any further bleeding or fever.

Incomplete abortion

Some of the products of conception, most frequently the placenta, remain attached to the uterine wall and are not expelled with the foetal component. If, after surgical removal of the retained products, the woman experiences bleeding several days later, she requires urgent medical attention, as hypovolaemic shock may ensue due to retention of tissue that was thought to have been removed during the surgical evacuation procedure.

Septic abortion

This is usually the result of an illegal attempt to procure an abortion by the use of non-sterile instruments to detach the foetus from the uterine wall, but may rarely follow incomplete abortion. The woman will develop a fever, abdominal pain (not usually described as contraction-like) and tachycardia. Sawaya *et al* (1996) found the most common causative pathogens to be *Staphylococcus aureus*, coliform bacteria and *Clostridium welchii*, but other bacteria may be present. There may be toxic shock from these organisms and the infection may spread to the pelvis, causing peritonitis, salpingitis (which has implications for future fertility) and septicaemia. The patient requires rapid hospitalisation and antibiotic therapy, including treatment for anaerobic organisms (e.g. cephalosporin and metronidazole; Sawaya *et al* 1996) which should be continued for a minimum of 5 days after temperature stabilisation. Uterine evacuation will be necessary as soon as the antibiotics have begun their beneficial action. The operation should be undertaken with great care, as the uterus is much more likely to perforate in the presence of infection (Rosevear 2002), and blood transfusion may be required. Syntometrine given intramuscularly will assist in haemostasis. There is a possibility of renal involvement and the nurse must carefully monitor urine output and in very severe cases of unresponsive septicaemia the uterus may have necrosed and require removal.

Missed abortion

This describes the situation when the embryo dies in the uterus and is retained in the gestational sac for some weeks. There is some blood loss into the choriodecidual space which eventually surrounds the dead embryo, causing it to separate from its placental attachment. The woman will probably notice some vaginal blood loss at around 10–12 weeks gestation, although this is not so in all cases. The breasts enlarge no further and eventually the woman, her midwife or her doctor will notice that the pregnancy is not progressing normally. The uterus is 'small-for-dates' and the cervix is closed. Diagnosis is confirmed by ultrasound, since immunological tests, which normally become negative 10 days after the death of the foetus, may confuse the diagnostician by remaining slightly positive for some time beyond the 10 days.

Missed abortions are usually expelled spontaneously, but this may not occur for some weeks and will cause great distress to the woman, who is aware of the non-viability of the pregnancy. To avoid some of this further anxiety, the uterus should be evacuated by suction curettage once diagnosis has been established.

The nurse must be aware of the confusion and sadness that the woman may be experiencing, and be able to offer the patient repeated explanations of the situation and support the woman and partner (if appropriate) through the stressful episode. Referral to a counselling service may be required, as the woman may be feeling guilty, since no cause for the death of the embryo is usually apparent.

Habitual or recurrent abortion

This refers to three or more consecutive spontaneous abortions before the 20th week of pregnancy. These can occur by chance; therefore no assumptions can be made regarding a single underlying cause unless the foetal losses have occurred at about the same gestational stage (Brigham *et al* 1999).

Habitual abortion is not common and affects about 1 in 200 couples or 1 in 500 pregnancies (Rosevear 2002). Women who subsequently conceive and continue the pregnancy to full term, have a high perinatal mortality rate due to an increased risk of sepsis and haemorrhage requiring very careful attention by the antenatal and delivery staff.

There is no 'absolute' treatment for women who have suffered from habitual abortion, except where a definite cause can be found and appropriate therapy instigated. Nevertheless, Stray-Pederson and Stray-Pederson (1984) devised Tender Loving Care (TLC) or stress-reducing empirical guidelines for management of recurrent pregnancy loss. These rules include over 20 quite stringent, stress-avoidance instructions such as:

◇ No exercise except walking for 10 minutes per day and swimming
◇ No weddings, funerals (except immediate family), dinner parties or house guests
◇ No travel
◇ Avoid crowds
◇ No sexual intercourse until 13 weeks or 2 weeks after gestation of previous loss. (The most likely time for recurrent abortion is 6–8 weeks.)

Maternal age appears to have an effect on the prognosis for future pregnancies. A 20-year-old woman who has experienced two spontaneous abortions has a 92% chance of success in a subsequent pregnancy, compared to a 45-year-old who has a success rate of 60% in similar circumstances (Clifford *et al* 1994).

Cervical incompetence is implicated in second trimester spontaneous abortions and is linked to trauma to the cervix. The cervix may be affected by any previously induced terminations of pregnancy, or by dilatation and curettage for investigation purposes.

The cervix dilates and there is spontaneous rupture of the membranes with uterine evacuation of a dead foetus. In some cases the cervix dilates and a viable foetus is delivered.

After one such abortion, early diagnosis can be established in subsequent pregnancies via ultrasonography and, where this occurs, the insertion of a Shirodkar suture which encircles the cervix in purse-string manner has resulted in a success rate of up to 90% (Lee and Slade 1996). This is performed at 14 weeks and the suture is removed at 38–39 weeks' gestation.

Criminal abortion

That which is carried out by persons unqualified to perform abortion or where it is carried out for other than legal reasons. Whilst the Abortion Act 1967 has dramatically reduced criminal abortions, they do still occur and do still cause morbidity and mortality in women.

Mortality following abortion

Chamberlain (1995) quotes figures from the Triennial Report on Confidential Enquiries into Maternal Deaths 1964–1966 indicating that 133 deaths occurred in England and Wales during those years, equalling 51.1 deaths per 1,000,000 maternities. Over half of those were from illegal terminations, in comparison to the 1985–87 figure of 6 deaths following abortion (2.7 per 1,000,000) in the UK as a whole. Of those six, only one followed legal intervention in the pregnancy, five occurred after spontaneous abortion, and there were no deaths from illegal terminations. The main cause of these deaths was sepsis.

Conclusion

Abortion is legally acceptable in Britain according to the Abortion Act 1967, amended 1990, but certain criteria have to be established prior to the termination of any pregnancy. The 1967 law was introduced in order to reduce the physical and psychological traumas experienced by women who had unwillingly become pregnant, or who found that their personal/family circumstances could not support a current pregnancy and its related future responsibilities.

Whilst there is no legal requirement for local health services to offer abortion facilities, most do, but the level of provision is variable, and in some areas private clinics appear to fill the service void at considerable cost to the woman requiring termination.

All service providers have to meet the legal requirements and be licensed to carry out abortions. They must fully complete all of the relevant documentation and forward it to the Department of Health within seven days of the termination having taken place.

Medical and surgical procedures are utilised at different stages of gestation according to the efficacy and likelihood of causing unwanted side-effects or later complications with fertility and pregnancy.

Nurses must recognise the physical and emotional implications for any female who undergoes a pregnancy termination, particularly as some of these may be young adolescents who are confused about their own sexuality and reproductive ability. There must be no intimation of guilt or reproach; each patient must be treated holistically and with respect as directed by the NMC (2002). Patient information must remain confidential and nurses should act as advocates where there is lack of knowledge, misunderstanding or misinterpretation of the facts or little trust in health care services.

Spontaneous abortions are usually traumatic events for pregnant women and nurses must be cognisant of the serious consequences to which the situation may lead. Excellent knowledge and skills, timely management and psychological support are essential for the woman and her partner in order to minimise the potentially traumatic effects that accompany this difficult situation.

Grieving is a natural process following a spontaneous abortion, but most women are also anxious to know why the pregnancy was lost and what the prospects are for future pregnancies. An open and honest explanation of current knowledge and an expected good prognosis for subsequent childbearing is likely to be helpful for the couple who have been traumatised by spontaneous abortion.

References

ASH (2001) *Smoking and Health Inequalities*. ASH, NHS Development Agency, London

Belfield, T (1999) *Contraceptive Handbook*. FPA, London

Brigham, S A, Conlon, C and Farquharson, R G (1999) A longitudinal study of pregnancy outcome following idiopathic recurrent miscarriage. *Human Reproduction* **14** 2868–2871

Chamberlain, G (1995) *Gynaecology*. Edward Arnold, London

Clifford, K, Rai, R, Watson, H and Regan, L (1994) An informative protocol for the investigation of recurrent miscarriage: preliminary experience of 500 consecutive cases. *Human Reproduction* **9** 1328–1332

Furedi, A (1996) *Unplanned Pregnancy – Your Choices*. Oxford University Press, Oxford

Kiddy, M (2002) Teenage pregnancy: whose problem? *Nursing Times* **98**(4) 36–37

Lee, C and Slade, P (1996) Miscarriage as a traumatic event: a review of the literature and implications for intervention. *Journal of Psychosomatic Research* **40** 232–245

Mahoney, C (1997) Abortion law matures. *Nursing Times* **93**(44) 12–14

Naidoo, J and Wills, J (2000) *Health Promotion: Foundations for Practice*, 2nd edn. Baillière Tindall, London

National Statistics (2003) *Social Trends*. HMSO, London

Nursing and Midwifery Council (2002) *Code of Conduct*. NMC, London

Rosevear, S (2002) *Handbook of Gynaecological Management*. Blackwell, Oxford

Sawaya, G, Grady, D, Kerlikowske, K and Grimes, D (1996) Antibiotics at the time of induced abortion: the case for universal prophylaxis based on a meta-analysis. *Obstetrics and Gynaecology* **87** 884–889

Spitz, I M, Bardin, C W, Benton, L and Robbins, A (1998) Early pregnancy termination with mifepristone and misoprostol in the United States. *New England Journal* **338** 1241–1247

Stray-Pederson, B and Stray-Pederson, S (1984) Etiological factors and subsequent reproductive performance in 195 couples with a prior history of habitual abortion. *American Journal of Obstetrics and Gynaecology* **148** 140–146

CHAPTER 3

The menopause

Introduction

This chapter is concerned with aspects of ageing and the quality of women's lives. It includes issues that are frequently related to the effects of the menopause (climacteric), such as the extent to which physical health or emotional problems interfere with normal work, daily activities and usual social interactions. Hormonal fluctuations and their short and long-term systemic effects are discussed, together with sources of help for the various symptoms that many women find distressing during menopausal years.

It would be useful for the reader to have a definitive understanding of the following:

◇ Menopause
◇ Perimenopause
◇ Climacteric
◇ Hormone Replacement Therapy (HRT)
◇ SERMS
◇ Amenorrhoea
◇ Body Mass Index (BMI)

However, these will all be discussed in the ensuing text.

The menopause

Throughout the world, women who live long enough will reach a stage in their lives when ovarian hormonal production declines and eventually stops. This process, if not surgically or medically induced, is gradual, occurring over a number of years, and as a woman approaches her late 40s the supply of ovarian follicles reduces, often with concurrent irregularity of the menstrual cycle or its complete cessation.

The combination of amenorrhoea and poverty of ovarian follicular activity is known as the *menopause* or *climacteric*, and is frequently referred to in lay terms as *the change*. It occurs on average in the UK at around the age of 51 years (Abernethy 1997).

Although the term 'menopause' literally means the last menstrual event, and is often used interchangeably with 'climacteric' and 'the change', many women associate the aforementioned menstrual and ovarian irregularities with a number of symptoms that present themselves over a period of months or years before and after the last menstrual period (Barclay 1997).

Before the menopause, the release of oestrogen from the ripening ovarian follicles is stimulated by rising levels of the pituitary secretion Follicle Stimulating Hormone (FSH) during the first half of the menstrual cycle. During the perimenopause, (approximately 1–2 years surrounding the actual menopause) oestrogen production is reduced due to smaller numbers of ovarian follicles being available for maturation. Consequently, the hypothalamus responds by increasing its output of Gonadotrophin Releasing Hormone (GnRH) in an attempt to achieve an increased production of FSH. The end result is very high levels of GnRH and FSH during this time, which may produce unwelcome symptoms and have a considerable impact upon a woman's quality of life.

Quality of life

There has been a growing awareness, particularly over recent years, of the aspects of quality of life and ageing. Direct questioning is a relatively easy way of providing information, albeit subjective, about how people carry out usual daily activities and how they feel, generally, in relation to becoming older.

It may be argued that psychological studies in relation to ageing have the potential to distress patients, but results from a study by Fallowfield *et al* (1987) indicated that the majority of patients value the opportunity to elaborate upon how symptoms and their control (or lack of) and treatment influence aspects of daily living.

Menopause is a critical physiological and psychological transition in a woman's life, and in the UK up to 80% of women reportedly suffer from associated symptoms. One in 3 of them classify their symptoms as 'severe', with 7% of women between 45 and 55 years consulting their general practitioner (GP) as a result (Barlow *et al* 1991).

However, Schneider and Dören (1996) highlight the fact that, according to 80% of women's own appraisals in their study:

Menopause occurs subtly, with no apparent loss in quality of life.

Additionally, 40% experienced a general improvement in well-being associated with the 'reliefs' of the menopause, these being greater personal independence following children leaving home and relief from pre-menstrual and menstrual problems, contraceptive mechanisms and pregnancy.

These may have been unexpectedly positive results due to the fact that the study concentrated upon the joy of living and quality of life aspects rather than negative menopausal symptoms.

Menopausal symptoms

Certainly, for many women, though by no means all, a reduction in quality of life is experienced from the fifth decade, with menopausal processes being associated with this decline. Many symptoms reported by perimenopausal women, according to Studd (2000), can be successfully managed providing a proper assessment has been undertaken and that women are encouraged to report at regular intervals the success, or otherwise, of management interventions.

A relatively simple classification of perimenopausal, menopausal and postmenopausal symptoms is the acute, medium and long-term situations as outlined by Abernethy (1997).

Acute perimenopausal/menopausal effects

Within this category lie those health problems most frequently complained of by perimenopausal women, which have a tendency to negatively affect family members and close friends. These include: unexplained anxiety, loss of confidence, emotional lability with crying outbursts occurring for apparently little reason, insomnia, irritability, tiredness without exertion, poor memory, inability to cope with relatively minor life difficulties that previously been dealt with easily, lack of self esteem, limited concentration span, hot flushes with visible skin reddening, night sweats (frequently commencing with a sudden sensation of warmth flooding the upper body, accompanied with a rise in skin temperature), tachycardia, and palpitations.

Many of the above 'vasomotor' symptoms would appear to be related to the excess levels of GnRH flooding the hypothalamic thermoregulatory system (Abernethy 1997), with which headaches, muscle pains and paraesthesia may also be related.

Medium/long-term effects

Osteoporosis

Osteoporosis is (Sturdee 1997):

> A systemic disease characterised by low bone mass and microarchitectural deterioration of bone tissue, leading to increased bone fragility and a consequent increase in fracture risk'.

For the first three years postmenopausally a woman can lose up to 5% of bone mass annually (Barlow 1994), subsequently, bone mass reduction slows down to about 2% annually. The significance of bone mass reduction postmenopausally is registered by the greatly increased risk of hip and wrist fractures when 25% of bone mass loss has been surpassed (Sturdee 1997).

Bone mass loss occurs for a number of reasons in both sexes, but after the peak of bone mass density at around the age of 35 years, it begins to decrease. When the rate of bone mass breakdown exceeds replacement, a steady loss of bone mass occurs which can lead to osteoporosis and the associated increased fracture risk.

In 1994, UK figures indicated that around 44,000 hip fractures were recorded annually, with an estimated financial NHS cost of £742 million (Barlow 1994), but the cost in terms of human suffering and death associated with hip fracture is inestimable.

According to Wyeth (2002), osteoporosis may be described as the 'silent epidemic', since so many people are affected by it, but most are unaware of their situation until they experience a fractured bone. Wyeth's (2002) statistics indicate that approximately 1 in 3 women and 1 in 12 men over 50 years of age are affected by osteoporosis, with over 200,000 fractures occurring annually.

Risk factors

For women, a reduced level of the female hormone oestrogen is the main contributory factor to osteoporosis (although not all postmenopausal women develop the disease), therefore the brittling of bones can be seen as a natural consequence of menopausal physiology.

However, factors other than natural menopause need to be recognised as potentiates to osteoporosis. Several of these are directly linked to oestrogen depletion and include:

◇ Early menopause (before age 45) induced by surgery, radiotherapy or chemotherapy, or medical conditions that cause endocrine imbalance.
◇ Premenopausal female reproductive tract surgery, when interference with ovarian blood supply adversely affects ovarian function, resulting in hormone secretion irregularity.
◇ Severe weight loss due to illness or over-enthusiastic dieting, which may result in menstrual irregularity and hormone disturbance

Matthews *et al* (1996) point out other risk factors, which include:

◇ Low Body Mass Index (BMI) – which may result in poverty of circulating oestrogen.

◇ Smoking – this is frequently linked to low BMI and low circulating oestrogen.

◇ Certain diseases that affect endocrine glands (e.g. thyroid over- or under-activity), which can adversely affect the total homoeostatic hormonal balance over which the pituitary/hypothalamic system maintains control.

◇ Some intestinal diseases that upset the absorption of minerals and vitamins.

◇ Liver disorders that disturb metabolism of nutrients and can have a significantly damaging effect on osteoblast activity.

◇ Prolonged bed rest or conditions that result in severely limited mobility with reduced blood flow, and hence the supply of nutrients required for bone metabolism are disrupted, leading to bone fragility.

◇ History of hip fracture in female relatives which may indicate an inherited tendency.

◇ Lifestyle contributory factors, such as limited exercise combined with smoking.

◇ Familial traits towards endocrine disorders.

Atherosclerosis

Evidence demonstrating links between loss of ovarian function and an increased risk of coronary artery disease is considerable (Sparkes 1991; Matthews *et al* 1996; Abernethy 1997; Meschia 1997).

Before the menopause, the incidence of myocardial infarction in women is about a third that of men, but after the menopause the incidence of coronary artery disease in women steadily rises, with post-menopausal women being at greater risk of arterial disease compared with premenopausal women of the same age (Gordon *et al* 1978).

The mortality risk from ischaemic heart disease for postmeno-pausal women eventually approaches that for men, and Darling *et al*

(1997) assert that cardiovascular disease is the leading cause of death in women over 50 years, accounting for over 50% of all causes and more than twice the level for malignant disease.

Risk factors

Those most at risk of medium to long-term consequences are women who:

◇ have suffered premature ovarian failure;
◇ have undergone early (before age 50) oophorectomy; or
◇ have had a hysterectomy, irrespective of removal of ovaries – ovarian failure is likely to occur at least 5 years earlier than the normal menopausal age due to disruption in blood supply induced by surgery of the reproductive tract.

Changes in lipid profile

Whilst the underlying mechanisms of increased risk of the aforementioned cardiac problems are not fully understood, the relationship between these and adverse changes in lipid profile has been well documented (Stampfer 1991; Van der Mooren 1993; Crook *et al* 1997). From these studies and, more recently, those undertaken by Webb *et al* (2000), it appears that the risk of heart disease is lower in people with high levels of high-density lipoprotein cholesterol (HDL) and low levels of low-density lipoprotein cholesterol (LDL).

Postmenopausally, the reverse begins to operate, where *total* levels of cholesterol, including LDL cholesterols, are increased, but HDL cholesterol concentration is reduced. Premenopausally, LDL cholesterol levels in women are generally lower than in men, but after the menopause LDL cholesterol levels in women rise above those in men (Van der Mooren 1993; Darling *et al* 1997).

The key issues related to atherosclerosis and lipid profiles changes postmenopausally can be summarised thus:

◇ The lifetime risk of coronary artery disease for a woman is around 45% (Grady 1992).

◇ Incidence of coronary heart disease in women increases postmenopausally.
◇ There is an increased atherogenic lipid profile in postmenopausal
women.

Changes in carbohydrate metabolism

The complex mechanism responsible for ensuring that levels of glucose in the blood remain at their optimum relates to the pituitary/hy-
pothalamic stimulatory and inhibitory effects upon the gonadotrophic
releasing hormone (GtRH), thyroid releasing hormone (TRH), thyroid
stimulating hormone (TSH), thyroxin, pancreatic hormones (insulin
and glucagon), liver function and glycogenolysis, the effectiveness of
the Krebs cycle, and the ability of the kidneys to filter, reabsorb and
excrete required or unrequired substances.

An understanding of this complex mechanism may be gained from
most human anatomy and physiology textbooks, but it is essential to
comprehend the interactions of endocrine and exocrine hormones.

Generally, unstable glucose control can occur through:

◇ Beta cells in the pancreas secreting insufficient insulin for the
body's requirements, resulting in Insulin Dependent Diabetes Mellitus (IDDM).
◇ Some resistance to the effects of insulin from the target cells. In
some people, where target cells have become resistant, glucose
accumulates in the blood resulting in Non-Insulin Dependent Diabetes Mellitus (NIDDM). In most people with insulin resistance,
however, this situation does not present, as the beta cells in the
pancreas respond by manufacturing and releasing more insulin.
Thus frank diabetes is not seen, but the patient develops chronic
hyperinsulinaemia as a result.

Stampfer (1991) found that the arterial deposition of lipids pro-
moted by insulin is compounded by sustained hyperinsulinaemia and
is therefore closely associated with the pathogenesis of atheroma. Ad-

ditionally, insulin resistance is frequently associated with other cardio-vascular risk factors, such as hypertension, reduced HDL cholesterol levels and obesity.

Postmenopausal oestrogen lack can result in reduced glucose tolerance and a gradual increase in insulin resistance. The contribution of insulin resistance towards the increase in coronary heart disease in postmenopausal women is not, as yet, firmly established.

The skin and urogenital tract

Collagen loss generally increases with the ageing process from the age of about 35 years, and this accelerates with diminishing oestrogen levels. This, over time, becomes more noticeable as thinner, less supple skin becomes drier and wrinkled. Many may regard the visible changes as mostly cosmetic, but the oestrogen-sensitive linings of the urogenital tract can present real problems for the postmenopausal woman. Indeed, Sturdee (1994) and Hope and Rees (1995) claim that up to 50% of postmenopausal women complain of vaginal dryness, loss of elasticity, dyspareunia, and frequency of micturition and incontinence related to hormone-depleted tissue atrophy.

Whilst population-based studies such as the Melbourne Women's Midlife Health project (Dennerstein *et al* 1993) suggest a downturn in aspects of female urinary tract activity associated with depleted hormone levels, it has to be recognised that several other factors are involved.

Continence is normally maintained by interaction of:

◇ Healthy urethral mucous membrane lining.
◇ Effective contraction and relaxation of voluntary and involuntary pelvic floor and urethral muscles.
◇ Appropriate relaxation of the bladder (detrusor) muscle at micturition

Thus hormone change is only one of several factors that influence urogenital functioning and Dennerstein *et al* (1993) argued that psychological and social issues also interact with the biophysical, particularly where urinary tract activity is concerned.

The brain

The growing population of people over 65 years old means that an increasing number will experience age-related psychophysical disorders such as stroke, Alzheimer's disease, anxiety and affective disorders, and a number of studies have made links between these neuropsychiatric disorders in women and reduced hormone activity (Phillips and Sherwin 1992; Burns and Murphy 1996; Doraiswamy *et al* 1997; Pedersen *et al* 1997).

One of the most disabling and distressing neuropsychiatric disorders – Alzheimer's disease – increases dramatically with age from around 1% at 65 years to about 15% of people in their 80s (Robertson *et al* 2000). It is accompanied by advancing memory loss and physical disability, causing immense impact upon sufferers and family members.

Stroke

Robertson *et al* (2000) note that the incidence of stroke in recent years has neither increased nor decreased noticeably, but the difference between fatal and non-fatal stroke, particularly amongst women, is more evident, with fatal stroke in females between 45 and 65 years being the third most common cause of death postmenopausally.

Neuropsychotic disorders

Hallonquist *et al* (1993) assert that women appear to have a greater preponderance over men towards particular age-related patterns of early/late onset of schizophrenia, symptomatology and outcome, and seasonal pattern. Harris (1997) links some psychiatric problems with peaks and dips of hormones that appear cyclically, in conjunction with the menstrual cycle.

Obesity

Whilst body weight tends to rise in both males and females with increasing age, the increase in women within their fourth and fifth decade is significant, and there are a number of predisposing factors suggested as relevant:

◇ Metabolic changes in lipid and glycoid nutrients
◇ Reduced thyroid activity leading to increased food intake
◇ Reduced physical activity, leading to lack of calorific utilisation

It is essential that the premenopausal increase in body weight be distinguished from obesity, the latter being noted as an excessive augmentation of body mass fat. Normally, fatty tissue represents between 20–25% of female body mass and is an energy reservoir.

The Body Mass Index (BMI) is a mathematical formula used to measure the degree of obesity in males and females, and calculated by dividing body weight in kilograms by the square of height (m^2). A person is considered to be overweight if the BMI is over 25 and obese if it is over 30, with indices of >26–27 being associated with increased risk of cardiovascular problems (British Nutrition Foundation 2001).

Age-related fat distribution in women tends to assume a similar upper body accumulation to men, which may provide an insight into the increasing incidence of heart attacks in postmenopausal women to that of the level of men.

Sexuality

Dennerstein *et al* (1993) noted the frequency with which women attending menopause clinics emphasised sexual difficulties, but there is a dearth of good-quality research into menopausal and postmenopausal women's sexual functioning.

Since hormone changes occur before, as well as during, the menopause, it would be necessary to study groups of pre- and postmenopausal women for evidence of sexual dysfunction, taking into account contributory and confounding factors.

The Melbourne Women's Midlife Health Project (Dennerstein *et al* 1993) was a longitudinal study that investigated the relationship between sexuality and a number of physical, psychological and social variables. The results suggested that the natural menopause was strongly linked to reduced libido and increased dyspareunia, but the deterioration in sexual functioning was also associated with factors such as general well-being, stress and partner problems.

Management of the menopause

The aim of treatment must be directed towards minimising the short- and long-term effects of hormone depletion without counterbalancing this by increasing unwanted effects to the level whereby a woman's general health is adversely compromised.

Hormone Replacement Therapy (HRT) was introduced to the UK before the Second World War, but subsequent improvements in education and the unwillingness to accept menopausal symptoms as inevitable have meant that it has grown in popularity as a treatment, to the extent that over a million women in this country are regular users of one or other type of preparation.

However, despite the demand for HRT, conflicting media reports and sometimes invalid research outcomes have caused confusion in the minds of many women, who are unsure as to the positive and negative aspects of its use (Brennan and Ayres 2003).

HRT is a group of drugs designed to work in a similar way to a woman's own reproductive hormones, thereby counteracting some of the symptoms produced by their natural depletion induced by the menopause.

Relief of acute symptoms

Porter *et al* (1996) menopause that the most commonly reported acute symptoms of the menopause are hot flushes (which occur nocturnally and disturb sleep), emotional lability, joint and muscle pains, reduced confidence, cystitis and irregular menses.

Oestrogen treatment

Oestrogen therapy began to be widely used with the development of orally active synthetic oestrogens, and the logic of their use is inescapable. Subsequently, methods have been developed to deliver natural oestradiol orally, by implant, topically (by transdermal patches) and by nasal spray.

When used as HRT, the actions of oestrogen are to:

◇ suppress the high levels of GnRH and FSH; and
◇ replace the falling levels of ovarian-produced oestrogen.

According to Purdie and Ballard (1996), psychological and vasomotor symptoms usually respond well to oestrogen therapy, as do vertigo, paraesthesia and muscular aches and pains, and the overall feeling of well-being is frequently improved. Indeed, Greendale (1998) argues that the above can be almost totally relieved by HRT.

Whilst the therapeutic aim of HRT is initially to relieve the acute symptoms of oestrogen deficiency, there is the twin objective of reducing the risk of medium- to long-term consequences of the menopause, which are sometimes fatal, as previously outlined.

Relief of medium- and long-term symptoms

Osteoporosis

Hextall (2000) contends that it is well established that prophylactic replacement of oestrogen can improve bone mineral density and reduce the number of osteoporotic fractures in postmenopausal women. Gordon *et al* (1978), in the Framingham Study, reported a markedly reduced incidence of hip fractures 30 years postmenopausally in women who had received oestrogen therapy at any time during those decades, and several further studies (Sturdee 1994; Kirby 1996), argue that all women at risk for osteoporosis should be considered for oestrogen therapy if there are no contraindications.

When oestrogen therapy is discontinued bone loss resumes; however, even users over 65 years of age show continued bone protection if they persist with oestrogen therapy. Delia (2003) suggests that HRT is also associated with improvement of symptoms in patients with rheumatoid arthritis.

Atherosclerotic changes in lipid profile

Numerous studies have indicated that postmenopausal oestrogen provides protection against CHD, reducing morbidity and mortality by between 25% and 50% in normal postmenopausal women and those with established CHD (Grady 1992; Matthews *et al* 1996; Purdie and Ballard 1996). There is also some evidence that oestrogen therapy has beneficial effects upon the lipid profile, reducing total cholesterol and LDL cholesterol whilst increasing HDL cholesterol (Darling *et al* 1997). When studying the effects of HRT on serum lipoproteins, it is important to understand the influence of the progestogen component of the regimen. (See progestogen information on pp. 97–98.)

Some progestogens used together with oestrogen may counteract the positive effects of oestrogen used alone, particularly in opposing the increase in HDL cholesterol.

Whilst several studies have indicated a strong correlation between HRT and lowered coronary heart disease due to reduced total cholesterol levels (Stampfer 1991; Gura 1995; Fuleihan 1997), the Women's Health Initiative (WHI) – a large study being undertaken in the USA and intended to continue until 2005 – was halted in 2003 as findings suggested that estimated primary and/or secondary prevention of heart disease may not be affected significantly by women's use of HRT. Indeed, the WHI study indicated that coronary heart disease risk in women taking combined oestrogen/progesterone HRT increased by 29%.

However, this signifies a very small increased risk overall and further evidence needs to be established in order to recommend use or non-use in relation to cardiac protection.

Changes in carbohydrate metabolism

Oestrogen replacement can improve the situation in relation to the impaired insulin response to glucose induced by oestrogen deficiency and progressive insulin resistance, but again, if combined oestrogen/progestogen is used, then the estimated reduction of overall benefits by some progestogens must be considered (Foster and Balfour 1997).

Skin and urogenital tract

Purdie and Ballard (1996) assert that, postmenopausally, women lose skin collagen at the rate of 2% each year for 15 years. This loss can be reduced but not stopped by HRT.

The impact of oestrogen on the once normal, but postmenopausally hormone depleted, urogenital system can be extremely beneficial. The main effect of the increased flexibility and softening of the urethral mucosa is improvement of the sealing of the urethral tissue layers (Sartori 1995).

There is also an increase in periurethral collagen elasticity, but the effect of this on continence is uncertain. However, a level of decreased detrusor muscle irritability would appear to be associated with reduction of urge incontinence (Versi 1994).

Generally, increased elasticity of periurethral tissues has the overall effect of improving symptoms of incontinence, with frequency, voiding difficulties and urinary tract infections all being reduced, thus giving the postmenopausal woman a much improved quality of life.

Bacterial urinary tract infection is a frequently reported female problem, with up to 10% of young women requiring treatment, and the incidence rises dramatically with age. Abruptyn *et al* (1988) note that up to 20% of 80-year-old women present with bactiuria. Several factors are associated with this situation, including incontinence, bladder prolapse and ineffective bladder emptying.

Their studies also indicated the potential predisposing factor of oestrogen depletion in postmenopausal women's development of urinary tract infections. The reduction in oestrogen is also associated with vaginal dryness, dyspareunia and pruritis.

Low oestrogen levels also cause reduction of the normal vaginal flora, which protect against enterobacteria. Enterobacteria such as

Streptococcus faecalis and *Escherichia coli* are frequently implicated in urinary tract infections.

In addition, the reduction of oestrogen causes loss of tone in vaginal muscles and hence pelvic floor ligament slackness, predisposing to cystocele and rectocele.

Raz and Stamm (1993) reported changes in vaginal flora following women receiving oestrogen either orally or vaginally, with an associated reduction in urge incontinence and urinary tract infection. There may, however, be carcinogenic side effects that require further research.

The brain and stroke

There are significant differences between male and female brain functioning processes (e.g. males' visuospatial functioning is superior to females, but females, when tested verbally, produce better results than males; Jarvik 1975). Cognitive abilities normally vary with the menstrual cycle in women who have not reached the menopause, with better articulatory and fine motor skills and sharper memory performance but decreased spatial ability during the first phase of the menstrual cycle (Phillips and Sherwin 1992).

Several early studies (Caldwell and Watson 1952; Feydor-Freybergh 1977; Campbell and Whitehead 1997) support the positive effects of oestrogen replacement therapy on women's memory and verbal ability, and more recently Resnick *et al* (1997) reported that oestrogen affects visual memory and new learning of visual presentations.

Oestrogen therapy is also associated with improved mood in healthy postmenopausal women. The study by Ditkoff *et al* (1991) indicated that the mood of postmenopausal women who took conjugated equine oestrogens improved significantly when compared with those receiving a placebo.

Generally, progestogens alter concentrations of chemicals in the brain and tend to antagonise the positive effects of oestrogen on mood, and have been associated with inducing depression (Dennerstein 1987). In depressive disorder, however, Oppenheim (1986) reported the positive effects of oestrogen therapy on 'mildly depressed' women, but similar treatment of 'clinically depressed' women appeared to increase the severity of the disorder.

There has been little evidence to suggest that oestrogen is useful as a treatment for depressive disorder, but it would appear that the HRT oestrogen doses offered to normal postmenopausal women are effective in improving mood.

With regard to Alzheimer's disease, oestrogens have reportedly very positive effects on the cerebral biological systems involved in this distressing condition. The study by Henderson *et al* (1994) reported significantly lower levels of Alzheimer's disease in women having HRT, and women with Alzheimer's disease receiving HRT had a more mild form of the disease than those who did not.

The study by Tang *et al* (1996) indicated that the risk of developing Alzheimer's disease is reduced by prolonged use of HRT and also delays its onset; in those women receiving oestrogen for more than 1 year, the risk of developing the disease reduces annually by 5%.

These interesting and exciting study outcomes do require further investigation, but the positive effects of oestrogen upon brain physiological processes cannot be ignored.

In relation to the risk for stroke, the case for hormone replacement therapy is less favourable and opinions conflict. Pettinin *et al* (1979) suggested that oestrogen therapy reduced the risk for women developing stroke, but Rosenberg (1980) reported a slight increase in this risk. Pedersen *et al* (1997) noted an increased risk in recipients of HRT compared with women who had never received therapy, yet Henderson *et al* (1994) had previously reported that the risk of stroke in women using combined HRT was significantly decreased.

Generally the current data suggest that present or past use of single dose (oestrogen) or combined (oestrogen and progesterone) HRT has little or no effect on the risk of stroke occurrence.

Neuropsychotic disorders

Given that gender differences in the development of schizophrenia suggest that hormone influences are protective against psychoses in the earlier years of women's lives, it could be that the reduction of oestrogen during the menopause is related to the higher hospital admission rates for female psychosis around the menopause. Riecher-Rossler *et al* (1994) found that women with schizophrenia appear to have lower oestradiol levels when compared with those without the disorder, but when women with florid symptoms were given oestrogen in conjunction with the usual antipsychotic drugs there was a slightly improved speed of recovery, but no definable improvement overall, in relation to antipsychotic medication without the oestrogen adjunct.

There is an obvious requirement for more research into this area of women's health, since depleted oestrogen levels seems to be implicated in many postmenopausal problems that women experience.

Obesity

Available data relating to the effects of HRT on obesity conflict (Reubinoff *et al* 1995) suggest that weight increase in postmenopausal women is not significantly influenced by oestrogen or combined therapeutic prescriptions. One extensive literature review (Tchernof *et al* 1998) asserts that most research suggests that HRT reduces the build-up of central body fat in postmenopausal women in comparison to control groups, but hypotheses need to be further tested against the variables.

The results of a study by Hanggi *et al* (1998) indicated that there was a difference in weight gain/loss between women treated by transdermal patch HRT and those using oral preparations. There may also be a familial factor as to weight gain/loss during the menopause; androgen levels decrease postmenopausally and this is know to have a genetic determination. Generally, the prevalence of obesity and the increase in its severity amongst UK adults does cause concern, and costs the NHS a minimum of £0.5 billion per annum in treating related disorders (Offer 2001).

Currently there is no evidence to either support or reject HRT as a more favourable influence over and above the control of calorific intake and taking exercise, in the management of obesity, pre- or postmenopausally.

Sexuality

Problems with loss of libido and vaginal atrophy postmenopausally, and subsequent dyspareunia, have been widely documented (Grady 1992; Raz and Stamm 1993; Sturdee 1994; Abernethy 1997). Women undoubtedly retain the desire to maintain attractiveness and libido during and after the menopause, but the reduction in circulating oestrogen levels causes, in many women, lethargy and thus an 'unwillingness' to participate in 'active' sexual intercourse.

HRT creams administered vaginally can produce relief of the local symptom of vaginal dryness and are generally useful for short-term effect; if longer-term relief is necessary then an additional progestogen oral preparation may be required.

Vaginal pessaries and also vaginal rings may be useful for local dryness. These are impregnated with oestrogen and are inserted into the vaginal crypt, releasing the hormone gradually over a 3-month period.

Purdie and Ballard (1996) reported that women complaining of urogenital tissue atrophy, which is likely to contribute to dyspareunia, have their symptoms rapidly relieved after commencing HRT.

There is also some evidence (Raz 1999) that the change in vaginal flora induced by oral/vaginal oestrogen reduced the incidence of urinary tract infections and urge incontinence postmenopausally. However, there may be potential carcinogenic implications, risk of thromboembolic disease and, in elderly women, the possibility of such physical limitations as obesity and tremor, when lower doses or oral estriol may have to be substituted.

Types of HRT

During the 1970s millions of women were prescribed oestrogen due to the perceived clear benefits in relieving climacteric symptoms. Commonly, oral oestrogen was given for 21 consecutive days, followed by a break of 7 days to allow for endometrial shedding (Sturdee 1994).

Reports of over-stimulation of the endometrium (endometrial hyperplasia), a pre-cancerous condition arising from incomplete endometrial shedding due to the lack of progesterone, appeared to be responsible for a six-fold increase in endometrial cancer in women who had used oestrogen for more than 5 years (Gambrell 1986).

By adding a progestogen to the regime, in order to transform the endometrium and promote complete shedding, it was found that the problem could be overcome. It was shown that 12–14 days of the correct dose of progestogen almost eliminated the risk of endometrial hyperplasia; this is known as 'opposed' therapy due to the opposing progestogen action (Gambrell 1986).

Various oestrogen forms are available:

◇ Synthetic oestrogens: these are compounds that have oestrogen-like action, but are chemically different structurally from oestrogens that women produce naturally. The most widely prescribed of these is ethinyloestradiol, mainly used in oral contraceptives due to its potency in suppressing GnRH and hence ovulation. It has, however, been implicated in causing the liver to produce elevated levels of blood clotting factors, thereby increasing the risk of thrombosis. It has also been implicated in increasing the amounts of renin substrate, which can lead to hypertension and its concomitant health problems.

◇ Natural oestrogens: this is the term given to any oestrogen compound, even if produced in a laboratory, that is very similar to the endogenous oestradiol that women naturally produce. The main ovarian oestrogen produced premenopausally is oestradiol, and this forms the basis of many types of HRT.

◇ Conjugated oestrogens: these are equine oestrogens extracted from the urine of pregnant mares. They contain a mixture of mainly oestrone and equilin, with variable amounts of dihydroequilin, sulphates and glucuronides. Sometimes confusion arises from them being labelled 'natural' in view of their animal origin.

Preparations

Local/systemic specific preparations

⟡ Vaginal creams, pessaries or rings are useful for relief of vaginal dryness and offer women some protection against urinary tract infections and urge incontinence.

⟡ Oral oestrogen or oestrogen–progestogen: a hysterectomised woman may be prescribed oestrogen-only HRT since uterine cancer is an impossible consequence, but oestrogen–progesterone combined therapy is needed for women with an intact uterus.

⟡ Topical/non-oral preparations: transdermal patches or gels are available, as are nasal sprays. These are not metabolised via the liver and therefore many of the side-effects of oral preparations, such as headaches, hypertension, nausea and dyspepsia, which may influence the woman's continuation with HRT, are avoided. Subcutaneous implants, which offer slow-release oestrogen (usually for 6 months), are available, but are used less frequently due to the need for minor surgery, discomfort and unsightliness complained of by some women, and difficulty in reversing side-effects. Progestogen needs to be taken by those women with an intact uterus. There are also reports of tachyphylaxis (a gradual reduction of dose response) which may necessitate an implant at decreasing intervals.

Progestogens

Since unopposed oestrogen use in postmenopausal women with an intact uterus is now contraindicated (Foster and Balfour 1997), several progestogens have been used to oppose the oestrogen effects in combined HRT regimes. The simplest classification subdivides them into those structurally related (chemically) to natural progesterone and those that are related to 19-nortestosterone.

Generally, short-term progestogenic side-effects include greasy skin, acne and disordered liver metabolism, but there are different longer-term effects.

The importance of the differing effects of the two main groups of progesterone on lipid profiles has a bearing on the long-term cardio-protective effects, where the 19-nortestosterone derivatives are more likely than progesterone to counter the desirable effects on the lipid profile, particularly on HDL-cholesterol (Crook *et al* 1997).

According to Gelfand *et al* (1997), dydrogesterone maintains the beneficial effects of oestrogen, whereas medroxyprogesterone acetate may reverse the beneficial effect when used at dosages sufficient to protect the endometrium.

Gelfand *et al* (1997) also suggest that there are differences between HRT regimens with respect to their effects on carbohydrate metabolism. Some oral HRT combinations of conjugated equine oestrogens with 19-nortestosterone progestogens have been reported to increase insulin resistance and impair glucose tolerance. There is some evidence that when medroxyprogesterone acetate is used in combination with conjugated oestrogens there is a slight increase in plasma glucose levels.

By contrast, long-term (24-month) studies have shown that a combination of oestradiol and dydrogesterone has no effects on glucose tolerance in postmenopausal women. Evidence suggests that this combination gave a substantial reduction in fasting insulin concentration, which may point to an improvement in insulin resistance (Crook *et al* 1997).

In summary:

◇ Progesterone derivatives tend to cause fewer androgenic side-effects than 19-nortestosterone derivatives.
◇ Progesterone derivatives are less likely to counteract the beneficial effects of oestrogen on an atherogenic lipid profile.
◇ Progesterone derivatives are less likely than 19-nortestosterone derivatives to alter glucose metabolism.

However, there can be differences between progesterone derivatives: dydrogesterone is beneficial to lipid and glucose metabolism, whereas medroxyprogesterone acetate is more likely to counteract lipid changes or alter glucose metabolism.

Alternatives to HRT

◇ No alternatives offer complete management of all menopausal problems.

◇ No alternative is free from side-effects.

◇ No alternative appears to reduce CHD in otherwise healthy individuals.

◇ No alternative currently exists that will reduce skin and urogenital atrophy.

◇ No alternative has been as widely researched in postmenopausal women.

The alternatives currently include medical, dietary and lifestyle interventions:

◇ Regular exercise such as aerobics, swimming and similar weight-bearing movements will reduce the risk of developing osteoporosis.

◇ Hypertensive symptoms that may induce hot flushes can be relieved by clonidine, but side-effects from this drug include nausea, insomnia, vertigo and dryness of oral mucosa.

◇ Tibolone, a synthetic hormone, is useful in the control of hot flushes, can improve libido and vaginal dryness and has the added advantage of mood enhancement. There is also some evidence (Prelevic *et al* 1996) of its ability to increase bone mass density of the spine and hip.

◇ Beta-blockers are useful antihypertensive drugs, thereby reducing the risk of stroke and cardiac disease postmenopausally, and can help relieve anxiety and panic attacks.

◇ Phytoestrogens (phytoproteins) are plant-based oestrogenic chemicals which are a common component of the far-eastern diet, found in such products as soya beans. Porter *et al* (1996) report that some of these phytoestrogens may delay and/or relieve menopausal symptoms.

◇ SERMs: these are a relatively recent group of compounds (Selective Estrogen Receptor Modulators) which characterise those drugs that can bind to and activate the oestrogen receptor, with distinctive tissue-specific effects. A SERM is a compound that produces oestrogen agonism in desired target tissues (e.g. liver or bone) together with oestrogen antagonism and/or clinically insignificant agonism in female reproductive tissue, such as uterus and breast.

  Tamoxifen and its derivatives were the initial representation of oestrogen-agonist properties in the endometrium, and have been successfully employed as a treatment for breast cancer. However, raloxifene, a second-generation SERM, has by contrast been developed as a prevention maintenance treatment for women post-menopausally. Useful in the prevention of osteoporosis in the post-menopausal situation, it is generating a great deal of interest as a potential preventative agent of breast and endometrial cancers (Brzozowski *et al* 1997).

◇ Bisphosphonates (formerly diphosphonates) are potent inhibitors of bone resorption and have been shown to offer a preventative and therapeutic approach to postmenopausal osteoporosis (Reginster 1996). Calcium and vitamin D supplements may be added to any of the above in order to prevent and treat osteoporosis.

◇ Black cohosh is a herb that may be used to treat menopausal symptoms and could be seen as a 'safe' alternative to HRT. The plant is of the buttercup species, and appears to act in the brain in a similar way to antidepressants by stimulating serotonin receptors. It had formerly been assumed that it mimicked the effects of oestrogen, but this has now been discredited. Ernst (2004) states:

  Previously, the criticism was that herbs act in more or less the same way as oestrogens and thus carry the same risks. This study suggests that this is not true.

  Black cohosh may therefore be an exciting addition to the therapeutic arsenal for menopausal symptoms in the future.

When HRT is inappropriate for menopausal problems

Some medical paternalists, such as Rymer (2000), seek to understand the difference between perimenopausal women who wish to assess the benefits of HRT via their GP and those women who do not consult a doctor.

It is impossible to make assumptions about the values of and reasons for women who do *not* visit their GP for advice as opposed to those women who *do* attend their GP surgery for therapeutic intervention.

Hartmann and Huber (1997) evaluated the HRT contraindications of five available oestrogen preparations and concluded that:

> The information in the pharmaceutical data sheets of HRT regimens should be modified, as it influences how these medications are prescribed by doctors, as well as affecting patient adherence.

This evaluation may be one reason, amongst many, that accounts for the compliance with or discontinuation of hormone replacement therapy by women so prescribed.

Research by Hunter *et al* (1997) suggests that women view very different criteria from their doctors when considering the use of HRT during their perimenopausal years, and there are also cultural aspects that need to be taken into account.

Rymer (2000) concludes that there is a small group of 'absolute' contraindications to the use of HRT preparations, these being:

◇ pregnancy
◇ acute venous thromboembolism
◇ active severe hepatic disease
◇ breast or uterine cancer

Additionally, some familial/pre-existing pathological conditions require serious consideration and investigation before prescription of HRT:

◇ abnormal vaginal bleeding
◇ family history of/personal pre-existing breast cancer
◇ uninvestigated breast lumps
◇ familial or personal history/high risk predisposition to thromboembolism
◇ history of endometrial cancer

There are also several disorders/diseases where caution prior to prescription of HRT is indicated:

◇ Diabetes mellitus: postmenopausally, there is a risk of increasing insulin resistance and increased insulin metabolism. These, combined with the decrease in insulin secretion, result in an increase in the overall levels of circulating insulin. In this situation, higher concentrations of circulating insulin are associated with raised blood lipids and may have an effect on atheroma development. Whilst perimenopausal women with diabetes could be encouraged to use HRT, they should be aware that its influence may require altered management of their diabetes.

◇ Liver and gall bladder disorders: since oral HRT is metabolised in the liver, alternatives should be offered to women who have liver and gall bladder problems.

◇ Uterine disorders: where previous endometriosis has been recognised, Rymer (2000) argues that prescribing HRT has not given rise to significant problems, but where there is concern, continuous combined HRT or tibolone might be preferred.

   In the case of a diagnosis of premenopausal fibroids, there is usually an expectation that these tumours will shrink postmenopausally as their dependent hormone, oestrogen, is reduced in the circulation. Offering HRT means that fibroid enlargement should be monitored regularly and HRT stopped if there is any undue increase in growth.

◇ Varicose veins: Jick *et al* (1996) assert that the presence of varicose veins doubles the risk of deep vein thrombosis post-operatively, thus women with varicosities who use HRT and who are likely to undergo surgery should be assessed, particularly if other predisposing factors (e.g. superficial phlebitis) coexist.

◇ Recent cardio/cerebrovascular disease: since periods of immobility which are likely to be induced by acute myocardial infarction or stroke can increase the risk of deep vein thrombosis (Autar 1996), HRT should be avoided during the acute immobilising stages and caution applied to use in the early rehabilitative period.

There are very few *total* contraindications to HRT, but there are a number where caution is necessary. Physicians and nurses need to comprehend the differences between oral contraceptives (which contain certain oestrogens and progestogens) and HRT, which are pharmaceutically similarly compounded, but because of the nature of their use are designed to achieve different outcomes. Some pharmaceutical data sheets tend to leave women unclear in this respect, and nurses have a duty to be able to give accurate and contemporaneous information.

It has to be accepted that in the concept of HRT, whilst adding both quantity and quality to the life years of postmenopausal women, there are areas of confusion – limited research and misinterpretation of results, particularly by news-hunting sensationalist media personnel who contribute to this situation.

The distressing symptoms of hot flushes, low and fluctuating mood, increased weight, sleeplessness and sexual problems tend to lead to the 'modern woman' (as opposed to those of yesteryear who simply 'put up with' such female difficulties) seeking assistance.

There is also a clear rise in osteoporosis and cardiovascular disease associated with the menopause (International Council of Nurses (ICN) 2001):

> Osteoporosis is responsible for 200,000 fractures every year in the UK, costing the NHS £1.6 billion.

Together, the acute problems and risks for diseases occurring later in life are widely accepted as being primarily due to the reduction in circulating oestrogen levels caused by ovarian decline, as characterised by the physiological female menopause (Brzozowski *et al* 1997; Hunter *et al* 1997; Delia 2003).

Oestrogen HRT is effective in the relief of many perimenopausal symptoms and has been shown to modify the above-mentioned risk factors. Some women may prefer to use alternatives to HRT; for some, HRT may be absolutely inadvisable; and others may be totally confused by media reports of 'bad news'.

In 1998 the North American Menopause Society Survey (Murphy *et al* 1998), asserted that, for the majority of menopausal women, midlife changes are viewed as positive in terms of life and health – these women therefore would not seek, nor want to use, HRT. The more recent study by Rabin *et al* (1999), involving 3000 women aged over 50 years, showed that almost half were not using any form of HRT. Of that number, 82% were experiencing the menopause, of whom 21% had previously been prescribed HRT.

The reasons described for *not* using HRT were:

◇ No longer experiencing the menopausal symptoms (49%)
◇ Not wishing to take HRT (45%)
◇ Not offered HRT by their family doctor (33%)
◇ Afraid of taking HRT (28%)

Therefore sometimes HRT use is not possible or available, which may be due to health care workers being less than active in pursuit of 'health promotion' and 'illness prevention'. Nevertheless, there are some situations that would indicate HRT as being very inadvisable, particularly for those women who have, or have had, oestrogen-related (reproductive tract) cancers and those with a strong family history of these tumours, until more conclusive research outcomes have been established. These include breast cancer (Sands and Studd 1995), uterine cancer (Chapman *et al* 1996), ovarian cancer (there has been a single review that reports outcomes in women who have been treated for ovarian cancers – Eeles *et al* 1991), and melanoma (Richardson 1995).

However, there are conflicting reports of an alleged melanoma risk among females using oral contraceptives (Beral *et al* 1977), and more recent evidence that premenopausal survival for women with melanoma is significantly greater than for those diagnosed postmenopausally (Jatoil and Gore 1993).

Probably the greatest concern for most women regarding HRT is the perceived and actual increased risk of breast cancer (Khastgir and Studd 1998). Most women of menopausal age will know or have known of other women who have developed this disease, and probably died as a result of its consequences. They may have witnessed the physiological and psychological pain and distress with which the disease is strongly associated (Richardson 1995), thus wishing to avoid any such similar situation for themselves, whatever the cost.

This is of course, completely understandable. However, if their perceptions reflected the truth of the situation in relation to other possible coincidental variables as previously discussed (e.g. hypertension, familial predisposition) then alarmist media reports might not be so destructive.

Three such reports occurred in 2003. One read (Maher 2003):

> UK clinical experts have advised that all HRT should aim to use the lowest effective dose, and be reviewed annually because of the risk of breast cancer.

and then proceeded to tell the general readers that:

> The benefit of symptom relief has to be offset against the **small** increase in the risk of breast cancer, cardiovascular disease and stroke.

Subsequently, a *Daily Mail* headline shouted (Hope 2003):

> Yet Another Risk with HRT

and warned women not to use HRT to prevent osteoporosis. This article followed advice to the UK government from the Committee on Safety of Medicines (CSM), that there would be no need to change a patient's HRT therapy immediately, but advised a review at her next appointment.

The advice was based on the 'Million Women Study', which was, in the same newspaper report, denounced by Professor John Stevenson of the British Menopause Society as being 'flawed' and its conclusions unsound. The report did not differentiate between drugs used through the menopause for the variety of symptoms of which women may complain, but simply clumped all prescriptions under the heading of HRT.

Whilst the article's main area of concentration was upon HRT and osteoporosis, it quoted Professor Stevenson as saying (Hope 2003):

> It has been known for some time that HRT is associated with an increased risk of breast cancer. But even in women taking HRT for ten years or more, the increase is only around 0.5 per cent, less than the increased risks associated with being overweight.

The following day, Hall (2003) (medical editor, *Daily Telegraph*), reported that Professor David Purdie had resigned from the Government advisory committee, the CSM, because of its decision to limit HRT due to perceived health risks. Purdie was adamant that general practitioners should still be able to prescribe HRT for osteoporosis prevention in women during their early fifties, stating that it is safe, reliable and effective, and had been responsible for a reduction of hip fractures by over a third in recent years.

Three further voices added to the conflict – Doctors John Stevenson and Margaret Rees, who both expressed surprise that the CSM should issue such advice:

> when there has been no long-term prospective study of the risk/benefit ratio for HRT given to women at increased risk of osteoporotic fractures.

However, Christine Fogg, of Breast Cancer Care, was reported as welcoming the CSM's advice. The above conflicting opinions do little to increase women's confidence in HRT use.

One major concern for GPs who prescribe HRT for their patients is non-compliance/early discontinuation of therapy. Domoney and Studd (1999) reported that there were several reasons for this, one of the most important being 'safety concerns'. Given the conflicting accounts of the value of HRT outlined above, it is unsurprising that women become confused and fearful of the therapy, which could dramatically improve quality and quantity of life.

Conclusion

HRT has been used for over half a century to improve the quality and quantity of women's lives peri- and postmenopausally. Much research into its actions and influences has given rise to fluctuating levels of uptake among the target group of women for whom it is designed and who are able to benefit from it, due to the misinterpretation of results of flawed methodology.

Many media headlines, expressed in a manner likely to engender huge caution and often fear in recipients, have contributed to variability in compliance and continuation.

There are definite benefits from HRT and certainly side-effects from its use. Several preparations are manufactured and women should not be discouraged from its use if one preparation appears to be unsuitable, before trying an alternative.

It is for the woman and her GP to decide whether or not HRT is appropriate and which preparation might be best for her.

Many GP practices now employ 'Menopause Nurse Specialists' who run clinics for women needing personal advice and information who may be reluctant to discuss intimate problems with their GP, and most large hospitals now run busy menopause clinics where specialist tests and investigations, such as bone densitometry, are carried out.

All nurses will come into contact with peri- and menopausal women who may seek information about this time of change in their lives. Many female nurses will experience some of its associated problems themselves and consider the various remedial options.

It is therefore vital that nurses maintain a working knowledge of current issues and therapies that continue to develop, so that they themselves and their patients, friends and family members feel confident in the decisions they may make for themselves.

References

Abernethy, K (1997) *The Menopause and HRT*. Baillière Tindall, London

Abruptyn, E, Biscia, J A and Kaye, D (1988) The treatment of asymptomatic bactiuria in the elderly. *Journal of American Geriatric Society* **36** 473–475

Autar, R (1996) *Deep Vein Thrombosis – The Silent Killer*. Quay Books, Wiltshire

Barclay, C S (1997) *Obstetrics and Gynaecology in General Practice*. Quay Books, Wiltshire

Barlow, D H (1994) *Department of Health Advisory Group on Osteoporosis Report*. Department of Health, London

Barlow, D H, Brockie, J A and Rees, M P (1991) Study of General Practice consultations and menopausal problems. *British Medical Journal* **302** 274–276

Beral, V, Ramcharan, S and Farini, R (1977) Malignant melanoma and oral contraceptive use amongst women in California. *British Journal of Cancer* **36** 804–809

Brennan, K and Ayres, J (2003) The pros and cons of hormone replacement therapy. *Nursing Times* **99**(35) 26–27

British Nutrition Foundation (2001) Coronary Heart Disease. http://www.nutrition.org.uk/

Brzozowski, A, Pike, A C and Dauter, Z (1997) Molecular basis of agonism and antagonism in the oestrogen receptor. *Nature (London)* **389** 753–758

Burns, A and Murphy, D (1996) Protection against Alzheimer's disease. *Lancet* **348** 420–421

Caldwell, B M and Watson, R I (1952) An evaluation of psychologic effects of sex hormone administration in aged women: Results of therapy after 6 months. *Journal of Gerontology* **7** 228–244

Campbell, S and Whitehead, M (1977) Oestrogen therapy and the menopausal Syndrome. *Clinical Obstetrics and Gynaecology* **4** 31–47

Chapman, J A, Berman, M L and Gillotte, D L (1996) Oestrogen replacement therapy in surgical stage I and II endometrial cancer survivors. *American Journal of obstetrics and Gynaecology* **175** 1195–2000

Crook, D, Godslad, I F, Hull, J and Stevenson, J C (1997) Hormone Replacement Therapy with dydrogesterone and 17β oestradiol: effects upon serum lipoprotein and glucose tolerance during 24 month follow-up. *British Journal of Obstetrics and Gynaecology* **104**(298) 3–4

Darling, G M, Johns, J A, McLeod, P L and Davis, S R (1997) Estrogen and progestin compared with simvastin for hypercholesterolaemia in postmenopausal women. *New England Journal of Medicine* **337** 598–601

Delia, H F (2003) Influence of hormone replacement therapy on disease progression and bone density in rheumatoid arthritis. *Journal of Rheumatology* **30**(7) 1456–1463

Dennerstein, L (1987) Depression in the menopause. *Obstetric Gynaecological Clinic, North America* **4** 33–48

Dennerstein, L, Smith, A and Morse, C (1993) Menopausal symptoms in Australian women. *Medical Journal of Australia* **159** 232–236

Ditkoff, E C, Crary, W G, Cristo, M and Lobo, R A (1991) Estrogen improves psychological function in asymptomatic postmenopausal women. *Obstetrics and Gynecology* **78** 991–995

Domoney, C L and Studd, J W (1999) Long-term continuation of hormone replacement therapy in hysterectomised women. Presented at the British Menopause Society meeting, Manchester, June 1999

Doraiswamy, P M, Krishen, A and Martin, W L (1997) Gender concurrent oestrogen use and cognition in Alzheimer's disease. *International Journal of Geriatric Psychopharmacology* **40** 34–37

Eeles, R A, Tau, S and Wilshaw, E (1991) Hormone replacement therapy and survival after surgery for ovarian cancer. *British Medical Journal* **302** 259–262

Ernst, E (2004) The case for black cohosh in the treatment of menopausal symptoms. *Journal of Agriculture and Food Chemistry* **46** 523–526

Fallowfield, L, Baum, M and Maquire, G P (1987) Do psychological studies upset patients? *Journal of the Royal Society of Medicine* **80** 59

Feydor-Freybergh, P (1977) The influence of oestrogen on wellbeing and mental performance in climacteric and postmenopausal women. *Acta Obstetrics and Gynaecology, Scandinavia* **64** 5–69

Foster, R H and Balfour, J A (1997) Estradiol and dydrogesterone: a review of their combined use as HRT in postmenopausal women. *Drugs and Ageing* **11**(5) 1–20

Fuleihan, G E (1997) Tissue-specific estrogens – the promise for the future. *New England Journal of Medicine* **337** 1686–1687

Gambrell, R D (1986) Prevention of endometrial cancer with progestogens. *Maturitas* **8** 159–168

Gelfand, M M, Fugere, P, Bissonnette, F, Wiita, B, Yang, H M, Lorrain J and Ferenczy, A (1997) Conjugated estrogens combined with sequential dydrogesterone or medroxyprogesterone acetate in postmenopausal women: effects on lipoproteins, glucose tolerance, endometrial history and bleeding. *Menopause* **4**(1) 10–18

Gordon, T, Kannel, W B, Hjortland, M C and McNamara, P M (1978) The Framingham Study. *Annals of International Medicine* **89** 157–161

Grady, D (1992) Hormone therapy to prevent disease and prolong life in post-menopausal women. *Annals of International Medicine* **117** 1016–1037

Greendale, G A (1998) Symptom relief and side effects from postmenopausal hormones: results from the postmenopausal estrogen/progestin interventions trial. *Obstetrics and Gynaecology* **92** 982–998

Gura, T (1995) Estrogen: key player in heart disease among women. *Science* **269** 771–773

Hall, C (2003) Bone specialist quits in protest at curb on 'safe' HRT. *Daily Telegraph* 5 Dec, p. 1

Hallonquist, J, Seeman, M V, Lang, M and Rector, N A (1993) Variation in the symptom severity over the menstrual cycle of schizophrenics. *Biological Psychiatry* **33** 207–209

Hanggi, W, Lippuner, K and Jaeger, P (1998) Differential impact of conventional oral or transdermal HRT or tibolone on body composition in post-menopausal women. *Clinical Endocrinology* **48** 691–699

Harris, A H (1997) Menstrually related symptom changes in women with schizophrenia. *Schizophrenia Research* **27** 93–99

Hartmann, B W and Huber, C (1997) The mythology of hormone replacement Therapy. *British Journal of Obstetrics and Gynaecology* **104** 163–168

Henderson, V, Paganini, A, Hill, A, Emanuel, C, Dunn, M and Buckwalter, J (1994) Estrogen replacement therapy in older women. *Archives of Neurology* **51** 896–900

Hextall, A (2000) Oestrogens and lower urinary tract function. *Maturitas* **36**(2) 83–92

Hope, J (2003) Yet another risk with HRT. *Daily Mail*, 4 Dec

Hope, S and Rees, C M P (1995) Why British women start and stop hormone replacement therapy. *Journal of the British Menopause Society* **1**(2) 26–28

Hunter, M S, O'Dea, I and Britten, N (1997) Decision making and hormone replacement therapy: a qualitative analysis. *Social Science and Medicine* **45** 1541–1548

International Council of Nurses (2001) ICN co-sponsors osteoporosis tour. *International Nursing Review* **48** 201

Jarvik, L F (1975) Human intelligence: sex differences. *Acta Genet Med Gemellol* (Rome) **24** 189–211

Jatoil, E and Gore, M E (1993) Sex, pregnancy, hormones and melanoma. *British Medical Journal* **307** 2–3

Jick, H, Derby, L E, Myers, M W, Vasilakis, C and Newton, K M (1996) Risk of hospital admission for idiopathic venous thromboembolism among users of postmenopausal oestrogens. *Lancet* **348** 981–983

Khastgir, G and Studd, J (1998) *Hysterectomy and HRT*. Dunitz, London

Kirby, M (1996) How can GPs stop bone loss? *Medical Monitor* **10**(7) 15–17

Maher, S (2003) Clinicians back use of low-dose HRT. *Nursing Times* **99**(41) 7

Matthews, K A, Kuller, L H and Wing, R R (1996) Prior to use of oestrogen therapy, are users healthier than non-users? *American Journal of Epidemiology* **143** 971–973

Meschia, M (1997) Effects of HRT on blood lipid and lipoprotein levels in 6834 postmenopausal women. Unpublished paper presented to the North European Congress on Menopause, Vienna, Austria (October 1997)

Murphy, D G M, Allen, G and Haxby, J V (1998) The effects of sex steroids and the X chromosome on female brain function: a study of the neuropsychology of adult Turner Syndrome. *Neuropsychology* **19**(32) 1309–1323

Offer, A (2001) Body weight and self control in the United States and Britain since the 1950s. *Social History of Medicine* **14**(1) 79–106

Oppenheim, G (1986) Estrogen in the treatment of depression: neuropharmacological mechanisms. *Archives of General Psychiatry* **43** 569–573

Pedersen, A T, Lidegard Ø, Kreiner, S and Ottersen, B (1997) Hormone replacement therapy and risk of non-fatal stroke. *Lancet* **350** 1277–1283

Pettinin, D B, Wingard, J, Pellegrin, F and Rancharan, S (1979) Risk of vascular disease in women: smoking, oral contraceptives, non-contraceptive estrogens and other factors. *Journal of the American Medical Society* **242** 1150–1154

Phillips, S M and Sherwin, B B (1992) Variations in memory function and sex steroid hormones across the menstrual cycle. *Psychoneuroendocrinology* **17** 497–506

Porter, M, Penney, G C, Russell, D, Russell, E and Templeton, A (1996) A population-based survey of women's experience of the menopause. *British Journal of Gynaecology* **103**(10) 1025–1028

Prelevic, G, Bartram, C and Wood, J (1996) Comparative effects on bone mineral density of tibolone, transdermal oestrogen and oral oestrogen/progestogen therapy in postmenopausal women. *Gynaecological Endocrinology* **10** 413–420

Purdie, D W and Ballard, P A (1996) *Non-gynaecological effects of hormone replacement therapy*. Review No 96, Royal College of Obstetricians and Gynaecologists, London

Rabin, D S, Cipparrone, N and Linn, E S (1999) Why menopausal women do not want to take HRT. *Menopause* **6** 61–67

Raz, R (1999) Role of estriol therapy for women with recurrent urinary tract infections: advantages and disadvantages. *Infectious Diseases Clinical Practitioner* **8** 159–168

Raz, R and Stamm, W E (1993) A controlled trial of intravaginal estriol in postmenopausal women with recurrent urinary tract infections. *New England Journal of Medicine* **329** 753–756

Reginster, J Y (2000) Les bisphosphonates constituent-ils un réal progrès thérapeutique dans l'ostéoprose? *Médecin Hygien* **54** 1497–1501

Riecher-Rossler, A, Hafner, H, Stumbaum, M, Maurer, K and Schmidt, R (1994) Can estradiol modulate schizophrenic symptomatology? *Schizophrenia Bulletin* **20** 203–14.

Reubinoff, B E, Wurtman, J and Rojansky, N (1995) Effects of hormone replacement therapy on weight, body composition, fat distribution and food intake in early postmenopausal women: a prospective study. *Fertility and Sterility* **64** 963–969

Resnick, S M, Metter, E J and Zondermann, A B (1997) Estrogen hormone replacement therapy and longitudinal decline in visual memory: a possible protective effect? *Neurology* **49** 1491–1497

Richardson, P (1995) *Nursing and Cancer.* Saunders, London

Robertson, D, van Amelsvoort, T and Murphy D (2000) In Studd, J (2000) *The Management of the Menopause: The Millennium Review.* Parthenon, Carnforth

Rosenberg, S H (1980) The role of estrogens as a risk factor for stroke in postmenopausal women. *Western Journal of Medicine* **133** 292–296

Rymer, J (2000) Relative and absolute contraindications to hormone replacement therapy. In Studd, J (2000) *The Management of the Menopause: The Millennium Review.* Parthenon, Carnforth

Sands, R H and Studd, J (1995) Exogenous androgens in postmenopausal women. *American Journal of Medicine* **98** 76–79

Sartori, M G (1995) Menopausal genuine stress urinary incontinence treated with conjugated estrogens plus progestogens. *International Journal of Gynaecology and Obstetrics* **49** 165–169

Schneider, H P G and Dören, M (1996) Traits for long-term acceptance of hormone replacement therapy – results of a representative German Survey. *European Menopausal Journal* **3** 94–98

Sparkes, S (1991) Hormone replacement therapy. *Practice Nurse Journal* **3** 567–572

Stampfer, M J (1991) Postmenopausal estrogen therapy and cardiovascular disease. *New England Journal of Medicine* **325** 756–762

Studd, J (2000) *The Management of the Menopause: The Millennium Review.* Parthenon, Carnforth

Sturdee, D (1994) Hormone replacement therapy: the benefits and the risks. *Prescribers' Journal* **34** 234–242

Sturdee, D (1997) Newer hormone replacement therapy regimens. *British Journal of Obstetrics and Gynaecology* **104** 1109–1115

Tang, M, Jacobs, D and Stern, Y (1996) Effects of oestrogen during menopause on risk and age at onset of Alzheimer's Disease. *Lancet* **348** 429–432

Tchernof, A, Calles-Escandon, J and Sites, C K (1998) Menopause, central body fatness and insulin resistance: effects of hormone replacement therapy. *Coronary Artery Disease* **9** 503–511

Van der Mooren, M J (1993) A 2-year study on the beneficial effects of 17β oestradiol-dydrogesterone therapy on serum lipoproteins and LP(a) in post-menopausal women: no additional unfavourable effects of dydrogesterone. *European Journal of Obstetrics and Gynaecology, Reproductive Biology* **52** 117–123

Versi, E (1994) The bladder in menopause: lower urinary tract dysfunction during the climacteric. *Current Problems of Obstetrics and Gynaecology* **17** 193–232

Webb, C M, Hayward, C S and Collins, P (2000) Changes in coronary arteries with oestrogen therapy. In Studd, J (2000) *The Management of the Menopause: The Millennium Review*. Parthenon, Carnforth

Wyeth UK (2002) *The Menopause and The Facts*. http://www.wyeth.co.uk/

Useful addresses and web sites

Age Concern
http://www.ageconcern.org.uk/

For Cancer Information and Support:
http://www.cancerhelp.org.uk/
http://www.cancerindex.org.uk/

Breast Cancer Care:
0808 800 6000

For osteoporosis advice and information:

National Osteoporosis Society
PO Box 10
Radstock
Bath
BA3 3YB

For complementary medicine guidance:

Institute for Complementary Medicine
http://www.Icmedicine.co.uk/
0120 7237 5167

CHAPTER 4

Infections and infestations

Introduction

This chapter discusses a number of common sexually transmitted diseases and related gynaecological conditions about which the nurse will frequently be quizzed by friends, neighbours, family members and patients. A degree of knowledge from the nurse will be expected by these inquisitors, therefore nurses should be able to respond positively to those questions and be aware of local advice and treatment centres to which clients may be referred.

Some of the implications of Sexually Transmitted Infections (STIs) have already been discussed in previous chapters, particularly in relation to infertility and spontaneous abortion, but more detailed exploration of the nature and effects of these infections will be offered in this chapter.

This section will not be discussing Human Immunodeficiency Virus (HIV) nor Acquired Immune Deficiency Syndrome (AIDS), since the huge amount of research into the nature and consequences of this infection is constantly updating knowledge with such rapidity that many texts are out of date almost as soon as they are published. Therefore the reader is directed towards the research articles that are frequently printed in reputable medical and nursing journals in order to expand knowledge.

Media headlines telling of 'STI explosions', although sensationalist in presentation, are not, on this occasion, exaggerated. The Health

Protection Agency (HPA) released figures in 2004 indicating a trebling of cases of STIs in England during the previous five years, with a registered number of 1.5 million (HPA 2004). All of the more well-known STIs showed increases of about 100%, with syphilis showing a huge peak of 716% increase.

Increasingly risky sexual activity amongst young people, and in particular gay men, has been blamed for this dramatic rise in STIs, but Hartley (2004) asserts that:

> As demand for sexual health services has increased so have waiting times, which causes delays in diagnosis and treatment.

While patients are waiting to be assessed in a genito-urinary medicine (GUM) clinic (and a recent survey by the Family Planning Association indicated waiting lists country-wide to be as long as 6 weeks) there is further risk of them transmitting their infections to other sexual partners.

Although the Department of Health launched a National Strategy for Sexual Health in 2002, extra funding to address this problem amounted to only £15 million, which resulted in some clinics having to reduce opening hours to less than 21 per week and having to cut sessions due to insufficient nurses training in this speciality. In addition, the Chief Medical Officer for England, Sir Liam Donaldson, argued in his annual report 'On the State of Public Health' (2003) that waiting times at GUM clinics were presenting 'a serious obstacle' to diagnosis and treatment of STIs, and urged that improvements should rapidly be made to avoid further massive increases in numbers.

Current statistics for STIs

From 1996 to 2001 the following increases were reported. However, many cases are probably unreported due to lack of symptoms or lack of awareness of the significance of symptoms.

◇ Gonorrhoea: 86%
◇ Chlamydia: 108%
◇ Syphilis: 500%

Theses alarming figures show no signs currently of receding, since figures from 2002–03 indicate further increases:

◇ Syphilis: 28%
◇ Chlamydia: 9%

These figures, published by Kelly (2003), were linked to inequalities in health generally; Kelly argued that:

> The inequalities in health repeat themselves in inequalities in sexual health

and that

> The highest burden is borne by women, gay men, teenagers, young adults and black and ethnic minorities.

The HPA (2004) published figures that supported Kelly's (2003) assertions, which showed that, in 2003, STIs in females in the 16–19 years age group were indeed a large proportion of the total recorded infections. For 2003 the statistics were:

◇ Gonorrhoea: 42% of females presenting were under 20 years of age, and many had a resistant form of the pathogen.
◇ Chlamydia: 36% of females presenting were under 20 years of age.

These figures indicating an increase of 24% in gonorrhoea cases and 20% in chlamydia cases over the 2001 figures in the age group.

Changing sexual behaviour, social deprivation, asymptomatic and resistant forms of infections, poor access to services and a degree of ignorance of risk factors were all implicated in the above statistics.

Tenant-Flowers (2004) presented figures from a study of 11,000 participants (1999–2000) which indicated that males reported between 8 and 12 sexual partners that year and women between 3 and 6 sexual partners.

She also reported that up to 14% of males have concurrent partners and females up to 9%. Both males and females in this study showed a reduction of age at first intercourse from 17 to 16 years and that there was an increased inconsistency of condom use. All of these factors point to an increase in the potential for sexually transmitted infections.

Sexually transmitted infections pose health risks for those affected in a number of ways. These include risks in pregnancy of low birth weight babies and an increase in the number of pre-term deliveries. There is also a strong possibility of pelvic inflammatory disease (particularly with chlamydia, which causes widespread pelvic adhesions) and infertility.

The newborn infant is at risk from several of these diseases, which may in fact be fatal in up to 50% in some cases.

Sexual health must be envisaged as a holistic approach to the emotional, physical, spiritual and sociological needs of each individual. Therefore nurses must respect that individuality and encourage patients/clients to seek appropriate health care and guidance that meets the distinctive requirements of each, as and when required.

The addresses of local and national GUM clinics/advice centres should be widely available, with nurses being able to reassure potential patients of confidentiality regarding attendance. This code of confidentiality can, however, cause problems, with individuals' general practitioners being unaware of a patient's sexual disease and being unable to follow up the GUM clinic's initial therapeutic input, resulting in further spread of the infective organism(s) – a dilemma exposed by Barton (2004).

Schools and universities are useful venues at which to advertise the local facilities, as are nightlife haunts, public houses and clubs where young people are likely to meet.

Management of STIs

One of the more difficult problems facing both medical and nursing staff working in the field of sexual health is history taking, as many patients will feel embarrassed and vulnerable on being asked to reveal very intimate personal details to a stranger. Some will not give their real name or address, but will offer a mobile phone number so that laboratory results can be texted to them, which makes tracing of sexual partners more difficult. Additionally, the population most at risk of STIs is young adults, which is also the group that is most likely to be involved with substance use (Health Education Board for Scotland 2000).

Hine (2001) shows a direct link between drug abuse and the conveyance of sexually transmitted diseases and, because of the illegal nature of drug trafficking, many young people might be concerned about having such links exposed if treatment for STIs is sought.

Good communication skills, using tact and discretion, are essential in order to help women and their partners feel reasonably comfortable during such interviews. The assessment should include biographical details with particular attention paid to the woman's obstetric history, spontaneous or planned abortions, sexual and contraceptive history and any urinary or other locally associated problems.

Chlamydia

Women presenting with any gynaecological pathology may also be carrying an asymptomatic infection. A particularly common pathogen – chlamydia – has been found to be the cause of endocervical infection in up to 37% of such patients (Smith and Kitchen 1994). This organism is the most common sexually transmitted infection, tends to have an incidence peak at around 20 years of age, and is associated with changes in sexual partners, women using the contraceptive pill and other non-protective sexual practices.

Barton (2004) announced that a probable 1 in 10 females in the city of London under the age of 24 years have chlamydial infection, which is frequently asymptomatic.

An asymptomatic woman may seek advice because her sexual partner does have symptoms, such as dysuria and abdominal pain. She may after some weeks develop similar symptoms – these are responsive to antibiotics – but if left untreated, or if a woman succumbs to subsequent chlamydial infection, ascending endometritis, salpingitis and general pelvic inflammatory disease may cause tubal problems leading to infertility in up to 50% of women. Tenant-Flowers (2004) reveals that the latency period for chlamydial infection is far longer than had been previously estimated, with a time span of up to 10 years being possible. This is an obvious cause for concern, as within that time many sexual partners may have unwittingly contracted the infection.

It is no longer acceptable for many patients to take erythromycin for 7–10 days, and the newer azithromycin single dose therapy is easy to prescribe and more acceptable for patients. As with any sexually transmitted disease, when *one* is diagnosed, it is entirely possible that *several* may be coexisting in the same person; therefore, investigations should not be limited to the suspected causative organism.

Bacterial vaginosis

This is a common infection caused by an overgrowth of intestinal micro-organisms in conjunction with a reduced level of vaginal lactobacilli, which would normally antagonise gut bacteria. Rosevear (2002) notes that the condition is frequently associated with medical interventions such as termination of pregnancy, hysterectomy and intrauterine contraceptive device insertion. Metronidazole is normally an effective treatment for bacterial vaginosis. Tenant-Flowers (2004) suggests a possible link with mycoplasma genitalium and bacterial vaginosis; both of these have been associated with cervicitis, endometritis and pelvic inflammatory disease, although Barton (2004) suggests that several different bacteria could be involved with vaginosis.

Potential infertility problems cannot be overlooked.

Candida albicans

This communicable disease, commonly known as 'thrush' is a yeast infection that causes intense itching around the vulva and a thick, white vaginal discharge. It is a common infection and is associated with the use of anti-biotics prescribed for other bacterial invasion, e.g. streptococcal upper res-piratory tract infections. Antibiotics tend to change the natural commensal vaginal flora that occur with cyclical oestrogen fluctuations.

Candida responds to antifungal agents and the drug clotrimoxa-zole is now available over the counter as a single vaginal pessary of 500 mg, which is usually effective. Women with this infection should be advised to withhold from sexual intercourse for two weeks, other-wise reinfection can occur (Rogers and Beardall 1999).

A few women (less than 5%) will develop chronic cyclical candidiasis, and may require more prolonged therapy over several months. However, Barton (2004) advises that recurrent candidiasis could be an early sign of HIV infection, which reduces the patient's normal immune response to infections of any kind. Such patients should always be offered HIV inves-tigations so that appropriate therapy can be arranged.

Trichomonas vaginalis

The causative organism of this sexually transmitted disease is a protozoan. It induces a malodorous, frothy, yellow/green vaginal discharge, but up to 50% of women may have no symptoms. According to Chamberlain (1995) and Rosevear (2002) this infection is frequently associated with other sexually transmitted diseases, particularly HIV and gonorrhoea, the latter having made an apparent comeback in the UK in recent years.

Both female and male partners require treatment with metronida-zole and they should be investigated for other sexually transmitted in-fections. It is known that *Trichomonas vaginalis* is increasingly becom-ing resistant to metronidazole, however; thus the patient may require therapy with a variety of drugs in order to overcome the infection.

Gonorrhoea

Gonorrhoea is a sexually transmitted disease caused by the Gram-neg-ative diploid bacterium *Neisseria gonorrhoea* (NG). Whilst the incubation period is 4–5 days, many infected people will show no symptoms and will therefore unwittingly be able to spread the infection via unprotected sexual intercourse. Midgeley (2002) reported a huge increase in this sexually transmitted infection since 1995: by up to 75% in both males and females, at a time that it was thought that gonorrhoea was virtually eliminated from the UK population.

Those most at risk are adolescents (Gilson and Mindel 2001); therefore there must be information directed at people in their teens and early twenties regarding the risk factors associated with contracting gonorrhoea. Whilst some may view a sexually transmitted disease as 'merely another infection', such as the common cold, it has implications for future fertility prospects that may not be appreciated at the time of infection.

Clinical presentations, whilst sometimes mythically thought of as symptomatic, are not present in up to 60% of those infected (Tenant-Flowers 2004), but may include purulent vaginal discharge, the causative organism of which may not always be detected by high vaginal swab.

Any vaginal discharge could be mistaken for usual cyclical vaginal exudate and mild lower abdominal pain/urgency/frequency of micturition associated with urinary tract infection. Thus a woman may ignore the discharge for many months, with obvious potential problems.

The potential problems related to symptoms that may go unnoticed include:

◇ sub-fertility due to low-grade pelvic inflammatory disease
◇ abscess formation in fallopian tubes or ovaries
◇ conjunctivitis

If a pregnant woman begins labour and has been diagnosed as currently infected with NG, the delivered child should be protected as much as possible from cross-infection. The baby will, as it descends through the vaginal exit, be in close contact with vaginal secretions and at high risk of being infected with the NG bacterium. Sadly, this may lead to visual problems in the infant if not speedily acted upon.

There is no one treatment to suit all. The organism must be tested for sensitivity to drug therapy, as its resistance changes within a few miles of each known NG positive locality. Tenant-Flowers (2004) indicates that in the whole of the London area in 2002, 11% of cases were resistant to ciprofloxacin and in 2002 King's College Hospital clinic data showed a resistance of 7% and St Thomas's Hospital clinic data a resistance of 5%. Thus treatment must be tailored to the individual.

Whilst for many ciprofloxacin 500 mg orally upon diagnosis is usually effective, if the organism is penicillin-sensitive, 3 gm ampicillin together with 1 gm probenecid orally may well be an effective combination, especially in the pregnant woman. Single treatments of cefixime or ciprofloxacin plus azithromycin can be given by health care practitioners where there is suspicion of gonorrhoea and where diagnostic delay would increase risks of further spread.

Some clinics have embarked upon cephalosporins for treatment where resistance to ciprofloxacin has spiralled, and where gonorrhoea, especially in large inner city areas, presents in epidemic proportions, as is currently the case in East London (Barton 2004).

Partners need to be treated at the same time, and where possible given antichlamydial therapy to reduce the risk of cross-infection.

Both partners should be advised that sexual activity should be avoided for the proceeding 10 days, and if either partner has not attended the genitourinary clinic for testing/treatment they should be encouraged to do so, as this is essential for their future sexual health.

Herpes genitalis

The herpes simplex virus (HSV) is a member of the Herpetovirinae group which is known to cause latent infection. The causative organism is usually transmitted through small tears in the genital or oral mucous membranes and will be excreted through genital or oral secretions for many years. This can pose serious problems for babies born to infected women – neonatal herpes can be fatal for affected infants, with infant mortality being at 50% and infant morbidity, according to

Tenant-Flowers (2004) being at a very similar rate. Thus Caesarean section may be offered to infected women in order to prevent neonatal mortality – nurses and midwives need to be aware of this serious potential problem.

The incubation period for the virus is between 1 and 3 weeks, but may be longer, and its symptoms could be confused with those of influenza and might therefore be given only minor attention.

However, the New Zealand HPV project (1999) indicated that severe dysuria and inguinal lymphoedema may feature, and urinary retention and severe perineal pain with proctitis have also been reported. Ulceration of the cervix, vulva, vagina and anus are early problems which can cause a profuse watery discharge, which is most unpleasant for the affected woman. Later problems include labial adhesions and pain of a degree that requires morphine-derived drugs for its control.

Treatment with acyclovir 1000 mg in divided doses for 5 days to control the virus is a frequent prescription and a local anaesthetic gel (such as lignocaine) may be necessary to prevent pre-micturition or pre-defaecation pain.

This group of viruses may cause meningitis and is also associated with spontaneous abortion and must be regarded seriously. Recurrent infection (depending upon the variant of the virus) is frequent. Rosevear (2002) indicates that, if HSV 2 is the causative organism the recurrence rate can be up to 90%, and for HSV 1 about 50% recurrence is likely.

What must be noted is that HSV:

◇ *is not* always painful
◇ *does not* always cause numerous ulcers – in fact a single sore is probably more common (Tenant-Flowers 2004)
◇ *will* stop causing symptoms eventually, providing immuno-suppression has not been involved

This infection is therefore not one to be ignored or treated light-heartedly.

Syphilis

This infection is caused by the *Treponema pallidum* spirochaete and usually causes a painless ulcer at the site of entry. These ulcers (known as chancres) can become infected by other pathogens, which may then cause pain.

Syphilis, along with other chronic infectious diseases, has a tendency to shroud its chronicity by appearing to lose the initial symptom(s) so that the infected person has no physical signs after a few days.

Unfortunately, after 28–45 days the 'secondary syphilitic' signs appear, with the infected person developing a rash, usually on hands and feet, mouth ulcers and flat, wart-like lesions in the genital area. If untreated, these symptoms and signs can continue for up to 4 years, and may be misdiagnosed as psychosomatic problems, low-grade viral infections or other disorders that might be considered as 'trivial'.

Tertiary (third-stage) syphilis develops after about 5 years of untreated infection and the patient may show signs of physical and mental disturbance (formerly described as General Paralysis of the Insane, or GPI), where problems of the nervous and cardiac systems combine to generate a distressing *choreic* situation. This is characterised by disorganised shaking movements and lack of coordination of mobility, eating and drinking, together with mental deterioration, which eventually leads to death.

Syphilis responds to antibiotic treatment at any stage, but as symptoms may be dismissed as a minor local or systemic infection, the host may not seek therapeutic intervention until serious neurological damage has occurred.

Genital warts

Over 150 different strains of the Human Papilloma Virus (HPV) have been identified and mostly given identification numbers. HPV 6–11 are benign and cause genital warts that usually respond to the application of podophyllotoxin, but this therapy is not advised for the pregnant woman, nor for those with very large wart clusters. Imiquimod 5% cream is an alternative that is proving to be very effective in treating introital and perianal warts, but again is inadvisable for use during pregnancy.

For the pregnant woman and for those with HPV who are not pregnant, cryotherapy is probably the safest and most effective treatment for genital warts, but unlike the aforementioned therapeutic applications, patients cannot self-administer this treatment and require a visit to the clinic or hospital and the use of local/general anaesthetic. Surgical or laser removal of genital warts may be an option.

Genital warts appear as single or multiple lumps around the vulvo-anal area that may resemble a cauliflower in appearance, or may be flat and almost unnoticeable within the labial folds.

If the warts are large this may indicate an associated candidiasis infection, and if they bleed or are particularly irritant, investigations may be required for localised malignant change, particularly vulval intraepithelial neoplasia.

Nurses must always be willing to spend time with patients explaining the problems associated with STIs, particularly those that have an oncogenic tendency such as HPV. They should adopt a non-judgemental approach, since if patients feel uneasy about divulging information to health care workers they are less inclined to seek help with these very versatile infections.

Infestations

Scabies

The female mite *Sarcoptes scabiei* is just visible to the naked eye, and burrows into the skin following close bodily contact with an infested person. When it infests the genital area, it can cause intense itching due to the trail of eggs and faeces deposited in the tracts so formed. The male is the smaller of the species and lives on the skin surface. The eggs develop into larvae in about 5 days (warmer conditions promote earlier hatching), and these larvae then tunnel sideways or upwards to nearby hair follicles, from which the adult mite emerges some 2–3 days later.

Whilst the genital area is often involved, due to the favourable prevailing conditions for transmission and growth, it is usually the hands, particularly between the fingers, that are initially infested.

Nurses involved in treating any such infested patient(s) should be aware of the stigma associated with contraction of the scabies infestation, in that few women wish to be viewed as 'unclean'.

The woman and any household contacts can self-treat topically with permethrin 5% cream or malathion 0.5% lotion. These need only to be applied from the neck down, as the mite does not affect the face, but the medicaments should be undisturbed for 24 hours following application.

Bed linen and clothing should be machine washed at high temperature (90 °C) and not reused for 2 weeks to avoid reinfestation.

There has been recent concern (Barton 2004) of scabetic resistance to the above medications. Therefore some clinics will be looking for alternative therapies for the scabies mite.

Pubic lice

The crab louse or *Phthirus pubis* is about 1 mm in length and attaches to pubic hairs, biting and extracting blood from the skin and thus causing extreme itching. White ovoid eggs can frequently be visualised attached to the pubic hair and sometimes adult lice are also seen.

One particularly diagnostic feature is that, on digital removal of a satiated louse, it will easily and audibly crush and release blood when squashed between *gloved* fingernails. Due to the need for universal precautions against cross-infection, any health care worker should never undertake investigative or therapeutic measures of any description where contact with another person's body fluids is a potentiality without appropriate protection.

As with all of the aforementioned infections, patients with either of these two infestations should also be screened for other sexually transmitted infections (WHO 1999).

Conclusion

The UK has witnessed a dramatic rise in the incidence of sexually transmitted infections and infestations since 1995. Obviously therefore, nurses working in gynaecological and sexual health situations will be presented with more people requiring assessment, advice and treatment regarding these problems.

There are significant new diagnostic and therapeutic developments which will assist health care workers in the fight against sexually transmitted diseases, but it is essential that nurses retain a holistic approach to caring for patients so diagnosed in order to avoid overlooking coexistent diseases that might be threatening to future health and life.

WHO (2000) suggested that childcare issues, problematic appointment systems and transport, all of which must be juggled with time management, can mean that many women who would be compliant with treatment schedules find it extremely difficult to do so.

Nurses must be able to respond positively to questions asked of them by women who have worries about possible sexually transmitted infections/infestations, and be able to enlighten them about local care provisions for sexual health problems.

Nurses must also maintain the human approach of sensitivity and compassion for which there is much respect amongst the general public. These aspects engender trust and a willingness to approach the 'knowledgeable doer' with individual concerns.

References

Barton, S (2004) Update on STIs. Unpublished paper presented to 'Advances in Gynaecology' Wolfsen Conference, November, London

Chamberlain, G (1995) *Gynaecology*. Edward Arnold, London

Donaldson, L (2003) *On the State of Public Health*. http://www.publications.doh/

Gilson, R and Mindel, A (2001) Sexually transmitted infections. *British Medical Journal* **322** 1160–1164

Hartley, J (2004) STI explosion demands urgent action. *Nursing Times* **100**(31) 6

Health Education Board for Scotland (2000) *Indicators for Health Education in Scotland: Summary of Findings from the 1998 Health Education Population Survey*. HEBS, Edinburgh

Health Protection Agency (2004) *HPA annual report.* http://www.hpa.org.uk/

Hine, D (2001) National perspective: United Kingdom. *Women's Health* **11**(4) 239–293

Kelly, M (2003) *Sexual Health and Health Inequalities*. House of Commons Select Committee Enquiry. DoH, London

Midgeley, C (2002) The price of casual sex. *The Times* 29 Jan, p. 8.

New Zealand HPV Project (1999) *Guidelines for the Management of Genital Warts and/or genital HPV in New Zealand*. HPV Project, Auckland, New Zealand

Rogers, C and Beardall, A J (1999) Recurrent vulvovaginal candidiasis: why does it occur? *International Journal of Sexually Transmitted Diseases and AIDS* **10** 435–441

Rosevear, S (2002) *Handbook of Gynaecological Management*. Blackwell Science, Oxford

Smith, J R and Kitchen, V S (1994) *Infection in Gynaecology*. Churchill Livingstone, Edinburgh

Tenant-Flowers, M (2004) Update on Women's STIs and HIV. Unpublished paper presented to 'Women's Health Issues' Wolfsen Conference, September, London

World Health Organisation (1999) *Laboratory tests for the detection of reproductive infections*. WHO Regional Office, Western Pacific

World Health Organisation (2000) *Women and Sexually Transmitted Infections*. Fact Sheet 249. WHO, Geneva

Useful websites

British Association for Sexual Health and HIV

http://www.bashh.org/

For National guidelines in managing all STIs and lists of all GUM clinics in the UK.

RU thinking

http://www.ruthinking.co.uk/

Web site that offers full information to sexually active teenagers and information about local services. Teenage Pregnancy Unit supports this site.

likeitis.org

http://www.likeitis.org.uk/

Reproductive health issues for non-professionals.

SEXplained

http://www.sexplained.com/

An accessible website which is aimed at young people and associated health care workers. Explicit 'Club Zone' included.

British Association for Sexual and Relationship Therapy

http://www.basrt.org.uk/

A list of therapists is provided on this web site.

CHAPTER 5

Common gynaecological disorders

Women frequently suffer from gynaecological conditions that may be minor and irritating or recurrent and persistent and very distressing.

This chapter addresses several of these disorders and suggest how an empathic approach by nurses can encourage women to divulge intimate details which could be advantageous when diagnosing and treating these gynaecological problems.

Those discussed are the more common ones, which are less life-threatening than such diseases as malignancy, serious haemorrhagic problems and known killers such as AIDS. Specialised texts covering HIV/AIDS and gynaecological cancers are widely available; therefore these topics, whilst briefly touched upon, will remain largely in the hands of those full-time specialists.

Closely related to the female reproductive tract is the urological system, which can be severely affected by gynaecological pathology. Some common urological problems will be mentioned in this chapter, but a more thorough urological assessment, together with implications for nursing practice and costs to the NHS will appear in Chapter 7.

It would be helpful for the reader to be able to define the following:

◇ Menarche
◇ Dysmenorrhoea: primary/secondary
◇ Endometriosis
◇ Fibroids/myomata
◇ Ovarian tumours – benign

These all appear in the text and will be explained. However, a good working knowledge of the anatomy and physiology of the female reproductive tract is a requirement in order to understand the information contained within this chapter.

Dysmenorrhoea

This may be defined as 'painful menstruation' and affects up to 95% of menstruating women at some time in their lives. In teenage women it is associated with frequent absences from school and employment (Jones 2004).

Since many nurses and part-time employees in industry are women this is likely to have a significant economic effect, but Gould (1998) argues that despite the distress that this condition causes to so many females, very few seek medical assistance, and therefore the frequency and intensity of the problem cannot be accurately recorded.

Gould (1998) asserts that nurses ought to be able to listen to affected women and explain the physiological processes of menstruation and some of the conditions that cause associated pain.

A 'usual' menstrual cycle is typically 28 days in length, but 25–32 days is considered normal and the process is controlled by pituitary and hypothalamic influences upon ovarian hormones (oestrogen and progesterone) and their subsequent local and systemic actions.

There are two types of dysmenorrhoea – primary and secondary.

Primary dysmenorrhoea

This usually occurs around the menarche (Proctor 2004b) where pain begins at or just prior to menstruation, is located in the lower abdomen, radiating to the thighs and loins, and is spasmodic in nature.

The pain usually lasts for between 8 and 72 hours, often accompanied by nausea and vomiting, visual disturbance and vertigo, which may lead to syncopal attacks (fainting); some women may experience associated diarrhoea.

Vance (1996) suggests that symptoms reduce in severity with age and may completely disappear following the birth of a first child.

Following ovulation (mid-cycle usually) the blood contains high levels of prostaglandins secreted by the uterus. Prostaglandins induce smooth muscle contraction, particularly of the uterus, but are rendered ineffective by the relatively high levels of circulating progesterone during the second half of the menstrual cycle. Progesterone levels fall significantly during this time if the woman is not pregnant, causing a rapid rise in prostaglandins, which in turn cause intense uterine contractions with endometrial shedding and varying degrees of dysmenorrhoea. Levels of both progesterone and prostaglandins vary cyclically between individual females and may change in individual women; therefore prediction of dysmenorrhoeic cycles is uncertain.

However, whilst this explanation may be correct for many women with primary dysmenorrhoea, Jones (2004) indicates that prostaglandin levels are not universally raised in women presenting with this problem.

For younger women, oral analgesia (if not nauseous), e.g. Ibuprofen, combined with topical heat application to the lower abdomen can be effective in relieving dysmenorrhoea, but not in its prevention (Cassidy 2001). The oral contraceptive pill (OCP) may be useful if non-steroidal anti-inflammatory drugs (NSAIDs) are ineffective, by inhibiting ovulation. The endometrial lining does not thicken to its potential under the influence of the OCP, resulting in reduction of the volume of menstrual flow, and therefore prostaglandin activity is less aggressive (Proctor 2004b).

Not all women, however, are able to tolerate the OCP, and for a few it is contraindicated. For a minority (10–20%) of women, the OCP, NSAIDs or combinations of both are unhelpful, and it may be that glyceryl trinitrate (GTN) transdermal patches could be effective.

Prescribed in this way, GTN relaxes uterine contractions, thus relieving menstrual pain. Pitroff (1996) explains that the benefit of this prescription is that, women can apply and remove the patches according to their individual symptoms, and thus it provides a degree of personal control.

Proctor (2004a) suggests that acupuncture can give relief from primary dysmenorrhoea and that for some women transcutaneous electrical nerve stimulation may be helpful.

Advice regarding the prevention of constipation may help some women, since a full rectum will resist the increasing pre-menstrual fullness of the uterine wall.

Locke and Warren (1999) note the general improvement in well-being and reduction of stress due to endorphin release from the brain. Endorphins increase pain thresholds and are produced more abundantly during exercise; therefore an improved exercise programme may contribute to a reduction of menstrual pain.

Secondary dysmenorrhoea

This is described as pain due to a detected primary cause, e.g. pelvic inflammatory disease, intra-uterine contraceptive devices, benign and malignant uterine tumours, and ovarian pathologies.

Pain is not limited to the menstrual cycle and usually begins some years after the menarche. It may be chronic in nature or alternate cyclically and may be associated with dyspareunia (Wolf and Schumann 1999).

A variety of investigations may be necessary before the primary pathological condition is diagnosed and treatment/nursing care aimed at resolving the underlying primary cause is established. Many of these investigations can be intimidating, uncomfortable and embarrassing for the woman, who has already suffered many indignities; therefore nurses must develop a genuine patient-centred approach, reflecting the needs of the individual woman requiring care.

Treatment and nursing care follows diagnosis of the primary cause, both of which are variable. Some of the remedies which help women with primary dysmenorrhoea will relieve symptoms of secondary dysmenorrhoea, including the increased ingestion of dietary fibre and regular exercise regimes combined with transcutaneous electrical nerve stimulation (Proctor 2004a), but there may be a need for surgical intervention where the primary cause is unresponsive to the above.

For a number of women, hysterectomy will be the only remedy for relieving secondary dysmenorrhoea (see Chapter 6 for details of this surgical intervention), but this is only undertaken as a last resort and where such a patient is absolutely clear that child-bearing is no longer one of her needs.

For most women, dysmenorrhoea is a condition that can be successfully treated, and nurses (being mostly female and viewed generally as approachable and knowledgeable regarding female reproductive system disorders) are likely to be consulted about this disabling problem.

It is obvious that nurses must be familiar with the anatomy and physiology of the female reproductive tract and comprehend the workings of the menstrual cycle in order to fulfil the role of health educator in relation to dysmenorrhoea.

Nurses should encourage women who suffer from this common, but greatly underestimated, gynaecological problem to seek professional help so that an accurate diagnosis and appropriate remedial therapy can be obtained in order to improve their quality of life and relieve the misery of dysmenorrhoea (Wolf and Schumann 1999).

Endometriosis

Endometriosis is one of the most common gynaecological conditions in women of reproductive age and is seen more frequently in nulliparous women, or those of low parity. It is also more common in women whose menarche commenced earlier than the average age, and it may have a familial tendency – but the cause remains obscure.

Normally, the endometrium proliferates during the menstrual cycle under the influence of oestrogen and progesterone in order to provide a secure implantation site for the fertilised ovum. If the ovum is not subsequently fertilised, the endometrium tears away from the myometrium and is shed together with approximately 50 ml blood, per vaginum.

Endometriosis is (Abdella and Rizk 1998):

> ... [the] presence of tissue, histologically similar to endometrium, outside the uterine cavity

Common sites for this displaced tissue are (Biley 1995):

◇ urinary bladder
◇ rectum
◇ around the ovaries
◇ scattered throughout the pelvis
◇ lungs
◇ breast
◇ nasal cavity

Several theories exist as to its cause, but it is known that endometrial cells migrate by a variety of methods from the uterine cavity into adjacent or distant tissues/organs. Abdella and Rizk (1998) suggest that these cells disperse by:

◇ Retrograde menstruation – as the lining is shed during menstruation, some endometrial cells are pushed down the fallopian tubes by the uterine contractions. The cells may then settle in the tubes or leave via the fimbriated ends and embed themselves in pelvic organs.
◇ Lymphatic dissemination – cells enter the lymphatic system and become entangled in lymph nodes or deposit themselves in lymphatic vessels.
◇ Vascular transmission – cells enter the blood stream and are transported around the body until they become obstructed by narrow vessels.
◇ Direct invasion – the endometrial cells may 'burrow' into the myometrium (adenomyosis).
◇ Misplaced embryological cells are activated by hormonal stimulation after puberty.

Wherever endometrial tissue is found in abnormal body sites, it behaves as though it were within the uterine cavity, growing throughout the menstrual cycle and tearing away from its host tissue during menstruation, causing bleeding.

As this blood cannot escape by its normal vaginal route, it will collect in the pelvic cavity or adjacent to abdominal/thoracic organs to which it has become attached, and over a period of several months blood-filled cysts will form which will enlarge over time. Such cysts may cause adhesions, pain and distortion and dysfunction of the organs affected (Garry *et al* 2000).

Signs and symptoms of endometriosis

Approximately 28% of women with endometriosis are asymptomatic (Sutton 1993), but most suffer from varying degrees of dysmenorrhoea, which often commences several days prior to menstruation at the time of ovulation. This causes pain specifically related to ovulation which continues until, and becomes more severe during, menstruation, with prolongation of menstrual bleeding and ultimately anaemia.

Rosevear (2002) notes that there is little correlation between the severity of symptoms and the spread of endometrial deposits.

Dyspareunia, pain on micturition and defaecation may also be featured depending on the sites of endometrial growth – backache is also a common symptom.

Abdella and Rizk (1998) report that endometriosis is a significant factor in women who request investigations and treatment for infertility. Endometriosis is implicated in female infertility for a number of reasons:

◇ Entrapment of the oocyte at ovulation, thereby preventing its entry into the fallopian tube.
◇ Mechanical obstruction of the fallopian tubes by the endometrial deposits.
◇ Distortion of pelvic structures, including fimbrial ends of the fallopian tubes, which fail to make contact with the released oocyte at ovulation.

◇ Some studies have indicated that women with endometriosis develop an increase in fluid volume that affects the motility of sperms and their ability to fix onto the zona pellucida of the ovum (Van der Linden 1996).

Diagnosis

Transabdominal and transvaginal ultrasound can readily detect endometriomas (tumours composed of endometrial tissue). ,However there may be some difficulty in differentiating between those masses and fibroids, cysts and myomata. Magnetic resonance imaging may prove to be more accurate in assessing the woman's pelvis when endometriosis is suspected, but conclusive diagnosis can only be made by laparoscopy.

Endometriosis is one of the most common benign gynaecological conditions and is almost always detected during a woman's reproductive years. Post-menopausal diagnosis of this disease is generally associated with hormone replacement therapy and only rarely have malignancies been found in the same area as ectopic endometrial deposits. Research to find links between endometrial deposits and malignant change has been inconclusive (Corson 1992).

Management of endometriosis

Management and treatment should aim to:

◇ make an accurate diagnosis
◇ identify the location and severity of endometrial disease
◇ provide symptom relief
◇ improve fertility prospects where these are affected

There are a number of treatment choices and their use depends upon the individual woman's needs. Treatment consists of medical or surgical interventions, or a combination of both.

Since the disease is progressively destructive in terms of distorting and causing dysfunction of pelvic and other organs, young women under 20 years of age who have a history of severe dysmenorrhoea unresponsive to analgesia should have laparoscopic confirmation of the disease prior to commencement of medical treatment – this is to prevent problems of later infertility. If infertility already exists and assistance is being sought, an early laparoscopy can help a woman to decide about obtaining assisted conception.

Medical therapy

For some women strong analgesia (e.g. dihydrocodeine) combined with NSAIDs and paracetamol may be effective, particularly where relaxation techniques can be used in association with the medicaments.

Endometriosis can be managed by the use of the combined oral contraceptive pill, which has fewer side-effects than the former regime. However, for women with fertility problems this is not a realistic option. Moderately high doses of progestogens appear to have a direct inhibitory effect on endometrial tissue, but also cause anovulation and reduced levels of oestradiol, which again would be unacceptable to the infertile woman.

A synthetic derivative of 17 α-ethinyltestosterone – danazol – can be used to create a pseudo menopause when prescribed for up to 6 months at a time. It suppresses ovulation and allows time for endometrial deposits to regress. Since it is androgenic, depending on dosage, varying degrees of side-effects may be experienced, including hirsutism, oedema, weight gain and deepening of the voice – the latter being irreversible. However, it is markedly effective in relieving pelvic pain, dysmenorrhoea and dyspareunia.

Women should be aware that, although anovulation is commonly associated with this drug, pregnancies have occurred, and if this is not wanted barrier contraceptive methods should be employed

Gestrinone is a synthetic steroid hormone, the use of which results in amenorrhoea and endometrial atrophy in a similar way to danazol. It has fewer androgenic side-effects, but again women should be advised to employ barrier contraceptive methods during its use (Abdella and Rizk 1998).

GnRH agonists lead to a reduction in pituitary function which suppresses ovarian steroid production and induces a pseudomenopause. Because there is greater bone loss with the use of these preparations than with a natural menopause (averaging 1% monthly during a 6 month treatment episode), with femoral neck and lumbar spine bone mineral density being significantly affected (and recovery not completely reversible), the therapy should only be prescribed for women who are resistant to other therapies and who need only temporary prescription (Van der Linden 1996).

Mifepristone (RU486) has been used to induce abortion, but also inhibits ovulation and suppresses bleeding from pelvic endometrial deposits. When used in doses of 100 mg daily for 3 months and 150 mg daily for 6 months, pelvic pain is reduced and a 55% reduction in endometrial implants has been found (Rosevear 2002).

Surgical treatment

Surgery is employed for both diagnosis and treatment of endometriosis. The use of surgical intervention depends upon the site(s) of the disease and the stage it has reached, together with the wishes of the woman to become pregnant.

It should:

◇ relieve symptoms of the disease
◇ remove endometrial deposits
◇ restore fertility where wanted
◇ prevent or delay progress of endometriosis

Surgical intervention may be undertaken by diathermy or excision of minor endometrial deposits when a diagnostic laparoscopy is performed and thus remove the need for further medical or surgical treatment.

Nevertheless, in women with mild to moderate disease, superficial removal of endometrial deposits by the use of ablative surgical methods has produced symptomatic improvement over a 6-month period (Sutton *et al* 1997).

During surgery, it is essential that all endometrial deposits are cleared, leaving the reproductive organs completely free from extra-uterine disease, especially in women wishing to have children.

The above usually results in resolution of the symptoms of the disease for the majority of women, with a 5 year risk of new endometriotic diagnosis of approximately 20% (Garry *et al* 2000).

For some women, where their pain has not been resolved by surgical intervention, a 'second look' laparoscopy may be appropriate. This will be considered for about 6–8 weeks after the initial intervention and will be designed to check for overlooked endometriotic deposits and to separate any new adhesions that may be forming. This 'second look' also enables the surgeon to assess the reproductive organs for fecundity.

At all stages, nurses must be aware of the patient's physical, psychological and social trauma and be willing and able through personal and professional knowledge to offer guidance and support to women who are dismayed and deeply concerned by the problems that their reproductive systems cause them.

Nurses must also be able to ensure the safety of patients about to undergo surgery by checking all of the pre-operative data including informed consent; to reassure women that they will receive appropriate care (and to ensure that this *is* the case); and to deliver a high standard of post-operative nursing care, with special regard to the patient's personal hygiene and maintenance of her privacy and dignity.

A useful guide for any nurse is to put her- or himself in the same situation where sexuality and reproductivity are the central issues of patiency, and ask themselves 'How would I like to be treated if this were me?'.

More radical surgery, e.g. hysterectomy with or without bilateral salpingo-oophorectomy, may be considered for women whose problems are unresponsive to the aforementioned therapies, or who do not wish to have children. For this type of surgical intervention, see Chapter 6.

Conclusion

Whilst both dysmenorrhoea and endometriosis are somewhat mysterious phenomena, several theories have contributed to an enhanced comprehension of the aetiology and pathology of these diseases.

The greater the willingness of women who suffer from them to approach nurses and medical practitioners for relief from or resolution of the associated traumatising symptoms, the more likely that these professionals will be encouraged to undertake research on the behalf of their patients.

Future research, when appropriately applied, will enable a greater positivity towards women's health in relation to these enigmatic diseases.

Fibroids

Fibroids are benign tumours composed of fibrous and muscle tissue. Myomas are similar in nature, but contain more muscle than fibrous tissue, the distinction being academic although the difference between the two can be detected by an experienced ultrasonographer. For the remainder of this section 'fibroids' will be taken to apply to both types of benign tumours.

The cause of fibroids is unknown, but they are very common phenomena occurring in up to 25% of women in the UK at post-mortem, many of whom would have been unaware of their presence since they were asymptomatic (Rosevear 2002).

Fibroids can occur singly, but are usually present in greater numbers and their size varies considerably (http://www.womens-health. co.uk/fibroids.htm). They are thought to be hormone-dependent, and if they cause no symptoms premenopausally, then after the menopause, when oestrogen and progesterone levels have depleted, fibroids shrink and generally become of no consequence.

It is known that fibroids are particularly common in obese women – which may be a response to the higher levels of circulating oestrogen

– and in women who are nulliparous or very athletic (Rosevear 2002). The latter two situations appear to contradict the high oestrogenic theory, since nulliparous women do not experience the high levels of circulating oestrogen of pregnancy, and the very athletic usually have very little of the adipose tissue which, when evident, increases oestrogen levels.

These relatively 'innocent' tumours, may develop in various areas of the uterus (Figure 5.1).

Intramural fibroids, growing within the uterine wall, are the most common.

Subserous fibroids grow between the perimetrium and myometrium and can become very large, causing pressure on adjacent organs. Fibroids may also develop between the myometrium and endometrium (submucosal), and at this position may contribute to infertility, but these are the least common.

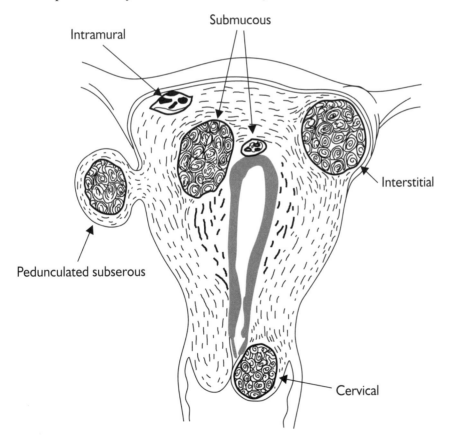

Figure 5.1: *Sites of uterine fibroids.*

Some subserosal benign tumours become 'pedunculated' and hang from the uterus by a stalk-like projection (pedicle) and may confuse diagnosis between fibroids and an ovarian tumour. Occasionally fibroids will develop in the cervix and cause dyspareunia.

Signs and symptoms

In many women fibroids are asymptomatic (Waugh and Grant 2001), but commonly dysmenorrhoea and menorrhagia are complained of. Large fibroids can cause pressure on and obstruct adjacent organs, resulting in abdominal discomfort, dysuria, defaecation difficulties and dyspareunia. Abdominal swelling may be the only symptom or sign that some women notice, but for younger women seeking pregnancy fibroids may be the cause of their infertility, depending upon their situation. Pedunculated fibroids may undergo torsion (twisting), causing acute abdominal pain, vomiting and circulatory shock. Emergency surgical intervention is required for this rare occurrence (Chamberlain 1995).

Diagnosis of fibroids

Diagnosis is confirmed by pelvic examination in association with the woman's reported signs and symptoms, together with ultrasound, or magnetic resonance imaging where ultrasound is inconclusive. It is usual to ensure that there is no malignant cervical pathology via a Papanicolaou smear analysis. A full blood count may show iron deficiency anaemia due to menorrhagia, and as with all gynaecological conditions experienced during reproductive years, pregnancy should be excluded prior to any surgical intervention (Chamberlain 1995).

Management

If a woman with fibroids is nearing the menopause and symptoms are minimal it is probably unnecessary to intervene medically, but nurses should be aware of the fact that women may approach them with questions about this common disease. Nurses need to be able to advise women who wish to become pregnant and who are experiencing difficulties due to fibroids that myomectomy via laser surgery is likely to resolve the problem – although fibroids do have a tendency to recur; thus the problem should be addressed sooner rather than later.

Contraceptive advice is often sought of nurses. Therefore they need to know that a woman with fibroids has a more limited choice than those who are fibroid-free. Intrauterine contraceptive devices are inadvisable as they may increase the severity of symptoms, and the oestrogen content of oral contraceptives might cause accelerated tumour growth. Depending upon the size and site of the fibroid(s) the use of a diaphragm contraceptive mechanism might induce dyspareunia (Rosevear 2002).

For many women, particularly those approaching menopause and who have no plans to have more children, hysterectomy may be the treatment of choice in order to reduce the potential damage to nearby organs, to reverse the anaemic effects of menorrhagia and to remove the distressing symptoms of pain, dyspareunia and other associated pelvic problems.

Whilst malignant change may occur, it is rare and is found in under 1% of women with fibroids (Rosevear 2002). Nurses should be aware that a rapid growth in the size of the diagnosed fibroid(s) accompanied by metrorrhagia signals the need for urgent reassessment and treatment of the affected woman.

A recently developed management technique is *uterine artery embolisation*, where a catheter is inserted into a small artery supplying blood to the fibroid. The catheter causes obstruction of the fibroid blood supply, with consequent shrinkage of the tumour.

Conclusion

Fibroids are common benign tumours occurring in women throughout the world. There are geographical and biological influences upon their development which are as yet uncertain in their degree and effect.

These tumours are usually innocent and may go unnoticed in many women, but being hormone-dependent they may gradually enlarge during reproductive life and generate problems both gynaecologically and within other pelvic organs. Post-menopausally they shrink and any associated problems diminish in severity.

Should surgery be advisable, its nature depends upon the age and reproductive wishes of the woman, and where hysterectomy is to be considered, the ovaries, if healthy, should be conserved and the reasons clearly explained to the patient.

Informed consent must always be confirmed before any surgical intervention of this nature so that the woman is completely clear of the consequences.

Benign ovarian tumours

The female gonads (ovaries) are situated in the pelvic cavity in close proximity to the fimbrial ends of the fallopian tubes and are held in position by the ovarian ligaments (Figure 5.2).

Often described as the size and shape of a walnut, each ovary enlarges at puberty and their former smooth, white surface becomes pitted and irregular due to scar formation following ovulation. Ovulation occurs mid-cycle under normal circumstances (in the absence of oral contraception or pregnancy) from the menarche until the menopause, at which time ovulation and menstruation cease and the ovaries become inactive and shrink.

Each ovary has a central medulla, composed of connective fibrous tissue that supports the outer cortical layer. The cortex contains the developing follicles, of which one or two will reach maturity and release its ovum midway through the menstrual cycle.

The ovaries are susceptible to sexually transmitted diseases and to benign and malignant tumours, but because they are positioned deeply within the pelvic cavity such conditions are difficult to diagnose in the early stages (Gould 2004).

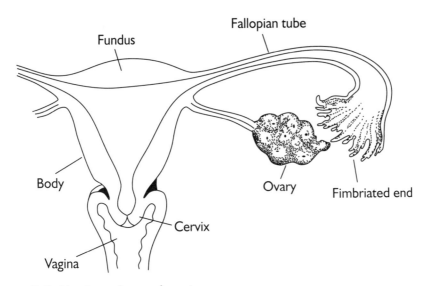

Figure 5.2: *Uterine tubes and ovaries.*

Very little is known about the causes and prevention of benign ovarian tumours and screening for them is rarely available. The ovarian cortex is physiologically active and is the site of origin of most benign tumours.

Ovarian cysts

These are fairly common phenomena and are associated with the cyclical endocrine activity of the organs. Some of these cysts develop in relation to endometriosis, and because they contain altered blood which becomes very dark in colour, they are described as 'chocolate' cysts (Gould 2003).

They are clearly visible on ultrasound investigation. Simple cysts may regress over time and do not need further intervention unless greater than 5 cm in diameter (Rosevear 2002). Larger cysts require further investigation due to the possibility of malignancy developing. Assessment of CA125, a cancer cell surface antigen, may be helpful in determining the likelihood of malignant change. The probability of malignancy increases with the size of the cyst, with 56% of cysts over 15 cm showing malignant change and 40% in the 5–15 cm group (Menon and Jacobs 2000).

The research undertaken by Vessey (1987) suggests that the use of the oral contraceptive pill, by preserving ovulation and follicular maturation, reduces the risk of ovarian cysts.

Ovarian cysts most commonly occur between the ages of 30 and 50 years, and:

◇ in the early stages are usually asymptomatic and are often discovered during an ante-natal ultrasound scan;
◇ often regress spontaneously, requiring no treatment;
◇ have the ability to undergo malignant change;
◇ may become large enough to compress adjacent organs, and may twist (torsion) or perforate.

Serous cystadenomas

This is the most common type of benign ovarian tumour diagnosed in women over 40 years of age. These cysts contain 'pockets' of clear, watery fluid and distend the surface of the ovary, giving it a smooth appearance rather than the pitted, scarred situation normally found. They are often asymptomatic as they do not grow very large, but can cause pain and discomfort if they perforate (Girling and Soutter 1997).

Mucinous cystadenomas

Between 16% and 30% of diagnosed ovarian cysts are of this type, which contain a thick fluid secreted by their mucus cell lining. They can become very large and occupy a major part of the peritoneal cavity. They may cause trauma to abdominal and pelvic organs from pressure, and may rupture.

Fibromas and Brenner tumours

These tumours are similar to the above in that they tend to develop in women over 60 years and are frequently bilateral. They consist mainly of fibrous connective tissue, may contain mucus and often grow to a large size.

Dermoid cysts

These are germ cell tumours and, unlike other cysts, usually occur in young women. Also known as 'benign cystic teratoma of the ovary', these cysts are seen at ultrasound to contain a solid component – the dermoid plug, which can be composed of various types of tissue such as teeth, bones and hair.

Such cysts are harmless unless they grow to a large size (causing local compression) or if they contain active tissue such as thyroid gland cells.

Occasionally, a large ovarian cyst can be misdiagnosed as pregnancy in a premenopausal woman, particularly if she has experienced related cessation of menstruation (Girling and Soutter 1997), but menstrual dysfunction is not a usual feature. X-ray and transvaginal ultrasound should aid diagnosis but may not be able to determine whether or not the cyst is malignant.

If ascites is present this is an ominous sign, but just because a cyst has become very large it does not indicate malignancy.

There are some tumours that may arise from the stromal area of the ovary and, although rare, they can secrete hormones that may cause a number of disturbing and distressing features. These include precocious puberty in young girls due to unusual oestrogen production and may result in early menarche and early development of secondary sexual characteristics.

Similar tumours develop from ovarian theca or granulosa cells in older women whose reproductive systems have matured. Such tumours can result in endometrial hyperplasia and associated metrorrhagia with tender breast enlargement.

More rarely, Leydig–Sertoli cells (which mimic those found in the male testicle), produce tumours that secrete androgens which will give rise to masculine features such as mammary atrophy, oligomenorrhoea, voice change and a more male distribution of body hair (Rose-vear 2002).

Management

Since benign ovarian tumours can become malignant, those over 5 cm in diameter or length require removal, which may take the following forms.

Ovarian cystectomy

This procedure is possible with fairly small tumours where malignant change is not suspected and where other trauma to the ovary that might have caused inflammatory responses and scarring has not occurred.

The tumour is extracted from its surrounding ovarian cortical capsule, which normally leaves ovarian function intact. Patients should be aware that this type of surgery does not mean that contraception is no longer necessary. Nurses should give appropriate advice regarding avoidance of pregnancy to women who have no desire to extend the family.

Resection

Where the cyst is small and there is minimal likelihood of carcinogenic change, a section of the ovarian cortex containing the cyst is surgically removed and the resulting cleft surgically secured.

Oophorectomy

If the size of the tumour has affected the function of the ovary or malignancy is a possibility, surgical removal must be undertaken.

It is usual to offer the woman a choice of unilateral oophorectomy and/or hysterectomy and bilateral salpingo-oophorectomy. When malignancy is confirmed, pre-operative radiotherapy/chemotherapy may be undertaken in order to shrink the tumour and enhance access to it with minimal blood loss during the surgical procedure.

The advantages of pre-operative interventions are:

◇ Metastatic spread may be limited, thus reducing the need for further post-operative intervention, either medically or surgically.
◇ Blood supply to the tumour is reduced, which in turn reduces the risk of haemorrhage.

Nursing implications

Many women who develop ovarian tumours may have little knowledge about their condition, which is unsurprising since little is known about benign ovarian tumours and predisposing factors to their development. Preventive measures are currently unknown, therefore health promotion relating to risk reduction is not possible. Benign ovarian tumours attract little media or research attention as they are not usually life-threatening.

Nevertheless, nurses need to be aware that any unusual abdominal distension that persists for more than a few days and increases in severity should be properly investigated, and they should be able to advise women that diagnostic procedures have been much improved during the last decade (Watson 2001).

Surgical intervention as a diagnostic procedure is now rare, and diagnosis can be concluded within a short time of ultrasound/blood testing procedures being completed.

Some women will naturally fear cancer of the ovary and may have read of or known others who have died of this disease. Thus nurses do need to show compassion and be willing to listen to fearful women and be able to explain the reasons for physiological changes that benign ovarian tumours may induce, e.g. hirsutism and menorrhagia.

Post-operative nursing care for those women who had required surgery needs to embrace an empathic approach, with nurses recognising that post-operative pain may be psychological as well as physical. Patients will require pain control in the form of medicinal analgesia, but also psychological care to reduce their anxieties.

Conclusion

Ovarian tumours vary in type – most are benign, but do have the ability to become malignant. Diagnosis can be difficult as many such tumours are asymptomatic and women may not notice, or attach any gravity to, their gradually increasing girth size or menstrual problems, which could be associated with the menopause, pregnancy or treatment for infertility.

When benign ovarian tumours become grossly enlarged, they may disturb the physiological processes of adjacent organs due to pressure being put upon them. This may give rise to symptoms suggestive of diseases of those associated organs and lead to unnecessary and unproductive diagnostic investigations.

Treatment aims to remove the affected tissue without compromising the woman's fertility, and nursing interventions involve the holistic approach of physical, psychological, social and spiritual care.

References

Abdella, H and Rizk, B (1998) *Endometriosis*. Health Press, Oxford

Biley, A (1995) Making sense of diagnosing and treating endometriosis. *Nursing Times* **91**(9) 33–34

Cassidy, M (2001) Dysmenorrhoea and puerperal pain. *The World of Irish Nursing* July/August 28–30.

Chamberlain, G (1995) *Gynaecology*. Edward Arnold, London

Corson, S L (1992) *Endometriosis: The Enigmatic Disease*. Durant, Canada

Garry, R, Clayton, R and Hawe, J (2000) The effect of endometriosis and its radical laparoscopic excision on quality of life indicators. *British Journal of Obstetrics and Gynaecology* **107** 44–45

Girling, K and Soutter, W (1997) Benign tumours of the ovary. In Shaw, R and Soutter, S (eds) *Gynaecology*. Churchill Livingstone, London

Gould, D (1998) Uterine problems: the menstrual cycle. *Nursing Standard* **12**(50) 38–43

Gould, D (2003) Endometriosis. *Nursing Standard* **19**(17) 47–53

Gould, D (2004) Benign ovarian tumours. *Nursing Standard* **18**(17) 45–52

Jones, A E (2004) Managing the pain of primary and secondary Dysmenorrhoea. *Nursing Times* **100**(10) 40–43

Locke, R J and Warren, M (1999) Exercise and primary dysmenorrhoea. *British Journal of Sports Medicine* **33**(4) 227

Menon, V and Jacobs, I (2000) Ovarian cancer screening in the general population. *Ultrasound in Obstetrics and Gynaecology* **15** 350–353

Pitroff, R (1996) Crossover study of glyceryl trinitrate patches for controlling pain in women with severe dysmenorrhoea. *British Medical Journal* **312** 884

Proctor, M L (2004a) *Transcutaneous electrical nerve stimulation and acupuncture for primary dysmenorrhoea.* The Cochrane Library: http://www.update-software.com/abstracts/AB002123.htm

Proctor, M L (2004b) *Combined oral contraceptive pill (OCP) as treatment for primary dysmenorrhoea.* The Cochrane Library: http://www.update-software.com/abstracts/AB002120.htm

Rosevear, S (2002) *Handbook of Gynaecological Management.* Blackwell Science, Oxford

Sutton, C (1993) Laser treatment of endometriosis. *Practitioner* **237** 601–607

Sutton, C, Pooley, A S, Ewen, S P and Haines, P (1997) Follow-up report on a randomised-controlled trial of laser laparoscopy in the treatment of pelvic pain associated with minimal to moderate endometriosis. *Fertility and Sterility* **68** 1070–1074

Van der Linden, P J (1996) Theories on the pathogenesis of endometriosis. *Human Reproduction* **11** 3–65

Vance, A R (1996) Microwave diathermy for primary dysmenorrhoea. *Physical Therapy* **15**(29) 47–53

Vessey, M (1987) Ovarian neoplasm, functional ovarian cysts and oral contraceptives. *British Medical Journal* **294** 1518–1520

Watson, H (2001) Polycystic ovary syndrome. In Ganger, E (ed) *Gynaecology: A Practical Guide.* Churchill Livingstone, Edinburgh

Waugh, A and Grant, A (2001) *Ross and Wilson Anatomy and Physiology.* Churchill Livingstone, Edinburgh

Wolf, L L and Schumann L (1999) C E Forum: dysmenorrhoea. *Journal of the American Academy of Nurse Practitioners* **111**(3) 125–132

Useful web sites

The British Menopause Society
http://www.the-bms.org/

Women's Health Information
http://www.womens-health.co.uk/fibroids.htm

National Institute for Clinical Excellence
http://www.nice.org.uk/
http://www.nice.org.uk/cms/ip/ipcat.aspx?o=56121

Family Planning Association
http://www.fpa.org.uk/

Wyeth UK
http://www.wyeth.co.uk/

Useful addresses

National Institute for Clinical Excellence
Midcity Place
71 High Holborn
London
WC1V 6NA

British Association for Counselling (BAC)
1 Regent Place
Rugby
CV21 2PJ
01788 578328

The SHE Trust
Red Hall Lodge Offices
Red Hall Drive
Bracebridge Heath
Lincoln
LN4 2JT
01522 519992

NHS Response line
0870 1555 455

CHAPTER 6

Hysterectomy

Introduction

This chapter introduces and addresses a very common surgical intervention – uterine removal – and will look at alternatives to this particular type of surgery.

Predisposing and potentially life-threatening factors that women and their gynaecologists might consider to be influential in the decision to proceed to hysterectomy are also included.

The nurse's role in helping women through what for some is a very traumatic period is included, and significant data are presented in relation to this surgery.

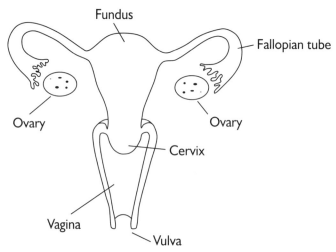

Figure 6.1: *Normal anatomy uterus, tubes and ovaries.*

The reader should be acquainted with definitions of the following in order to comprehend the text. However, explanations will be found within the chapter.

◇ Uterus
◇ Salpynx and salpingectomy
◇ Ovary and oophorectomy
◇ Hysterectomy
◇ Adenomyosis
◇ Fibroids/myomas

Hysterectomy

Removal of the uterus (or part of the organ) (Figure 6.1) may be performed for a number of pathological conditions. The organ may be removed via an abdominal incision, via laparoscopy or vaginally depending upon the pre-existing pathology, and may be accompanied by unilateral or bilateral oophorectomy and salpingectomy. The woman's menopausal history and her personal choice as to which type of surgical intervention she would prefer should also be considered.

As with many health problems, trends and treatments change with new insights provided by results of contemporaneous research. In gynaecology particularly, reduced parity, improved management of the woman in labour and the introduction of hormone therapies as alternatives to hysterectomy for menorrhagia have led to a reduction in the number of these operations during the past two decades.

Hysterectomy is still, however, the most commonly performed gynaecological surgery (Rosevear 2002). This may be performed via an abdominal incision or laparoscopically (depending upon the prevailing pathological condition). All options and procedures must be fully explained to any woman who is likely to be offered this major surgical procedure as a potential cure for her gynaecological problems.

Whilst most surgical procedures have an improving mortality rate year on year, there are risks attached to all of them. Mortality for hysterectomy is about 9:10,000 operations, with morbidity ranging between 3%–42% (Scottish Hysteroscopy Audit Group 1995).

Reasons for hysterectomy

The woman's wish for or ability to reproduce must always be considered in any situation where hysterectomy is judged to be beneficial. The outcome *must* be the best balance for that woman seeking medical and nursing care, and the type of surgery must be suited to the woman's age and presenting pathology.

Endometriosis and fibroids (adenomyosis) may be resolved by hysterectomy, providing the woman does not wish to conceive in the future. If the ovaries are unaffected by any disease they may be left intact; however, research by Namnoun *et al* (1995) indicates that over 10% of women with conserved ovaries at hysterectomy require further gynaecological surgery within the following decade due to pathological disorder affecting those conserved organs. This is often cyst formation, which is not life-threatening but does cause considerable discomfort and pain that might have been avoided by oophorectomy at the time of hysterectomy. This needs to be explained to women who opt for ovarian preservation when hysterectomy is performed (Clarke *et al* 1995).

Where utero-vaginal prolapse is present, approximately 7% of women choose hysterectomy – the majority of these women are post-menopausal, and therefore childbearing is not an issue.

Up to 6% of women with reproductive tract cancer will be offered, and benefit from, hysterectomy, which may be combined with chemotherapy and radiotherapy plus removal of ovaries (oophorectomy).

Occasionally, emergency hysterectomy may be essential to preserve the life of a woman, post-partum, who haemorrhages uncontrollably and for whom no other treatment is effective. This is an extremely difficult situation for the woman, her family and nurses and midwives caring for her, as it is usually the first (and last) pregnancy when this complication arises.

Types of hysterectomy

Vaginal or Laparoscopic Assisted Vaginal Hysterectomy (LAVH)

According to Rosevear (2002), many more vaginal hysterectomies versus abdominal hysterectomies are potentially within the ability of most surgeons. Vaginal hysterectomies are inadvisable where uterine size exceeds a 14 week pregnancy and where uterine mobility is restricted, e.g. by adhesions to other pelvic/abdominal organs. Where malignancy is suspected, or where there are chronic inflammatory or genetic anatomical abnormalities, vaginal hysterectomy is equally contraindicated.

Advantages include:

◇ Women invariable recover more quickly than from abdominal surgery, due to the fact that there is no abdominal incision. Consequently post-operative pain is neither severe nor protracted in comparison.

◇ Early mobilisation is much more likely and eating and drinking resume more quickly than with TAH (see below), with the result that urinary tract infections diminish in number and severity (Wilson and Bourcler 1999).

◇ Cosmetically, the results of vaginal hysterectomy show no indication of external scarring (but this does not mean that internal adhesions will not develop and become a future problem). For many women this effect may be a significantly influential factor in the type of treatment that they choose to be appropriate for their particular situation.

◇ Post-operative complications, such as Deep Vein Thrombosis (DVT) or chest infections, are less likely to develop, due to earlier, more comfortable post-operative mobilisation (Chamberlain 1995).

Total Abdominal Hysterectomy (TAH)

Indications for TAH (Figure 6.2), with or without removal of either or both fallopian tubes and ovaries, depend upon the prevailing pathology that necessitates surgical intervention.

Some women with fibroids who are peri-menopausal and are experiencing menstrual problems may choose TAH; others with the same difficulties at a similar time of life might prefer to 'ride out' the symptoms and let nature take her course.

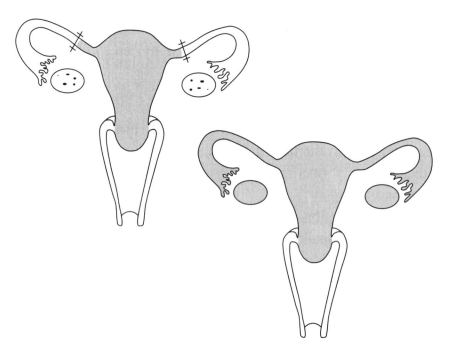

Figure 6.2: *Total hysterectomy and total hysterectomy with bilateral salpingo-oophorectomy.*

Fibroids usually diminish in size and symptom production post-menopausally, and the associated problems self-resolve.

In the case of cancer of the uterus, fallopian tubes, ovaries or fibroids that have reached a diameter of over 15 cm, TAH with bilateral salpingo-oophorectomy (TAH + BSO) would normally be the treatment advised. In this instance, the uterus, both fallopian tubes and the ovaries are excised. Menopausal symptoms would occur almost immediately when ovarian function is no longer present.

For most women undergoing a hysterectomy, few problems will be encountered. Whilst the procedure can be completed in about one hour by a skilled surgeon, it is still regarded as major surgery and nursing preparation must be thorough, with pre-operative check-lists adhered to rigorously.

Nursing implications

Particular attention should be paid to women who have been using the contraceptive pill pre-operatively, as there is an increased risk of thromboembolic disease during and after major surgery if the pill is not discontinued three weeks prior to surgery (Autar 2003). Thromboembolic deterrent stockings should be available for all women who are about to undergo major abdominal surgery.

Fasting prior to surgery is essential in order to prevent post-operative inhalation of regurgitated gastric contents. However, nurses must act on behalf of patients in order to prevent unnecessary post-operative dehydration from prolonged pre-operative fasting. Several authors have indicated from their research (Hung 1992; Maltby 1993; Jester and Williams 1999; O'Callaghan 2002), that nurses, despite knowing that patients physiologically need only to be fasted between 4–6 hours pre-operatively, frequently starve them for between 10 and 12 hours – generally because nurses were instructed to do so by doctors, or because theatre lists are changed and ward staff are not informed of the alterations. Here is a major area in which nurses should be using their research-based knowledge to effect change that will benefit patients.

Post-operatively, as with any surgery where a general anaesthetic has been employed, maintenance of the patient's airway and monitoring of respiratory function and circulatory status is essential. Blood pressure should be monitored and recorded at 30 minute intervals for a minimum of 2 hours and continued until stable. If blood pressure fluctuates dramatically or continues to be lower than would normally be expected (generally in the range 140/60–170/80) then the medical team should be alerted. Pulse rate is also recorded and should be within the normal 60–80 beats per minute range. Again, if this varies widely or if the pulse becomes erratic, thin and thready, or difficult to establish, medical expertise should be sought. The nurse will also observe the patient's skin and conjunctiva for signs of hypoxia. This can be clearly seen in white-skinned people by a blue tinge to the extremities and pallor of the conjunctivae, but in non-white-skinned patients it is necessary to look at the palms of their hands for signs of hypoxia. Most hospital wards now have oximetry devices that measure blood oxygen saturation levels and will alert nurses to the fact that the patient is having respiratory difficulties causing impairment of cellular oxygenation, and they in turn will inform medical staff of the situation.

Analgesia is frequently administered by the anaesthetist before the patient is roused from the anaesthetic, and fluid balance is maintained via an intravenous line. The nurse must maintain pain control and this may be done by assisting the woman with a 'patient-controlled analgesic system' or 'pcas'. The system gives the patient confidence in managing her own pain intravenously, without the risk of accidental overdose. Once the intravenous analgesic system is no longer needed, slow-release analgesia in the form of rectal suppositories (e.g. diclofenac) or oral paracetamol may be all that is required to keep the patient comfortable. However, strong analgesia may cause constipation and nurses need to be aware of this potentiality.

Sometimes a urinary catheter is inserted into the urinary bladder where trauma to the urethra may have occurred. Subsequently oedema of the perineum could cause retention of urine, which the catheter will overcome. Nurses should monitor urinary output in order to detect retention of urine at an early stage, so that catheterisation can be instituted as a relief measure if necessary, and should monitor vaginal blood loss. The latter should diminish with time and usually lasts no longer than ten days post-surgery (Wyeth 2000).

The intravenous line will be removed as soon as the woman is eating and drinking adequately. Nurses will offer the patient mouth care until she is able to drink sufficiently to maintain hydration levels.

The wound may be closed by subcuticular continuous thread, staples or clips which can be removed by the community nurse in the patient's home if she is discharged before complete wound healing. In hospital, the nurse will check the wound frequently for haematoma development, infection or haemorrhage. In some cases there may also be a wound drain to manage. Drains are normally removed when drainage is less than 50 ml per 24 hours – nurses must record drainage accurately.

The patient is encouraged to mobilise as soon as possible after surgery (12–18 hours) and to practise deep-breathing exercises in order to prevent deep vein thrombosis and chest infection. The elastic stockings with which the patient will have been fitted pre-operatively, are worn post-operatively for several days to avoid deep vein thrombosis and the surgeon may have prescribed prophylactic heparin where there is a concern relating to this potential (Autar 2003).

One very important nursing aspect both pre- and post-hysterectomy is the psychological support of the patient. Many women view their reproductive tract as the epitome of femininity and womanhood and may feel less of a woman and therefore unattractive to their partner as a result of hysterectomy. Nurses must be willing to address these issues and to let the patient know that hysterectomy should not interfere with sexual intercourse, although it is advisable to abstain for 6–8 weeks post-operatively until a follow-up examination confirms that internal healing is complete.

The operation should not affect libido. In fact, many women find that the freedom from menstruation, no further need for contraception and the impossibility of pregnancy make sexual activity more enjoyable. Some women may not realise that menstruation will cease and this should be made clear to them, as should the fact that oophorectomy will result in the onset of menopausal symptoms, but that hormone replacement therapy (see Chapter 3) can be prescribed to modify these (Wyeth 2002).

Many women fear weight increase after hysterectomy (Clarke *et al* 1995) and should be advised that the operation in itself does not induce this. Often, though, because they feel better in themselves, they may eat more than previously, causing calorific imbalance.

The nurse has a health education role in relation to advising about a balanced diet and regular exercise – swimming is a particularly helpful form of exercise in improving muscle tone, as is walking.

Most women are discharged home between 4–7 days after TAH, having suffered no complications. Continuous care advice should be available in written form and in appropriate language, to which women can refer once home.

A very small number of women do develop complications and Clarke *et al* (1995) found that:

◇ 5.2% developed a wound infection
◇ 5.0% developed a urinary tract infection
◇ 5.5% developed other infections
◇ 3.8% had some excessive bleeding
◇ 1.4% developed deep vein thrombosis or pulmonary embolism

and that:

◇ approximately 1% suffered operative bowel injury
◇ up to 2% suffered operative bladder injury
◇ 0.05% suffered operative ureteric injury.

Rosevear (2002) also reports that previously present psychiatric disturbance may be worsened by hysterectomy, but normally the evidence indicates a general improvement in mood following this surgical intervention.

Radical hysterectomy/Wertheim's hysterectomy

This major and quite devastating surgery is usually reserved for cervical malignancy and may be accompanied by chemotherapy and/or radiotherapy, depending upon the histology of the tumour and the extent of spread.

This extensive surgical procedure (see Figure 6.3) was introduced in the early 20th century as (Jordan 1989):

> [the] complete resolution of gynaecological misfortune

and was carried out on women with a variety of minor and major uterine conditions. It left women with no uterus or ovaries and a very short vagina – which meant no hope of child bearing or pleasure in sexual activity.

Thus it is only now carried out in the most necessary circumstances and involves removal of the uterus, fallopian tubes, ovaries, the parametrium and paracolpos, the upper one third to a half of the vagina and the pelvic lymph nodes, including the common iliac nodes (Lee and Flynn 2000).

It was thought that cure rates for radiotherapy and surgery were similar in early stage malignancy, but that surgery had some advan-

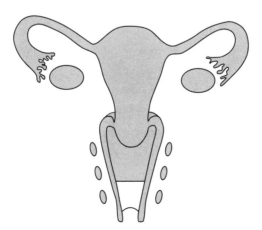

Figure 6.3 *Wertheim's hysterectomy.*

tages in that pelvic spread could be more accurately assessed and left the patient less debilitated and with less trauma to surrounding tissues and with the possibility of ovarian preservation in younger patients (Kurman *et al* 1992). However, recent research (Thomas 2000) has indicated the advantages of chemotherapy plus irradiation for cancer of the cervix.

Subtotal hysterectomy

This surgical procedure was fairly common in the mid-20th century for some decades (Chamberlain 1995), and involved removal of the body and fundus of the uterus, while preserving the cervix (see Figure 6.4).

Improved research (Kurman *et al* 1992) showed that the stump of the cervix left *in situ* was just as likely to develop malignant change as an intact uterus and that fibroids can develop in this remnant of reproductive tissue.

Treatment results for cancer of the cervical stump are much worse than that for an intact uterus, since radiotherapy is considerably more difficult to deliver with accuracy and without trauma to the bladder

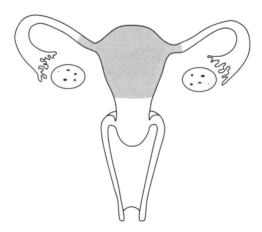

Figure 6.4 *Subtotal hysterectomy.*

and bowel, and further surgical intervention is troublesome due to the initial operation having left scar tissue and distorted surrounding anatomical support tissue.

Chamberlain (1995) states that:

> Stump carcinoma is an avoidable disaster. With very rare exceptions, there is no justification for the performance of subtotal hysterectomy in any patient who has had intercourse.

It has, however, become an increasingly observed entry onto recent gynaecological operative lists, as media reports appear to have influenced women's decision-making by suggesting that minimal surgical intervention of the female reproductive tract preserves libido and sexual satisfaction.

Women *do* have the right to make decisions about types of medical/surgical treatments to which they wish to submit, but nurses also need to have the knowledge and ability to ensure that their gynaecological patients make decisions that are fully informed and appropriate to the individual's circumstances.

Conclusion

Hysterectomy is a frequently performed surgical intervention for both benign and malignant reproductive tract conditions. It may or may not be accompanied by removal of one or both fallopian tubes and/or ovaries.

A number of different techniques may be employed, depending upon the predisposing pathology, age of the woman and desire for delaying menopausal symptoms.

It may be necessary to undergo combined treatments in the case of malignancy (although this aspect is only briefly discussed in this chapter – further information may be gathered from Johnson (2004)) and the nurse's role relates to helping women accept body image alterations and reducing potential post-operative complications. Health education is important as women may feel that hysterectomy could have adverse effects upon their future potential, and as new research findings are presented, nurses must be able to appraise them critically and press for their implementation when patients are likely to benefit.

References

Autar, R (2003) The management of deep vein thrombosis: the Autar DVT risk-assessment scale revisited. *Journal of Orthopaedic Nursing* **7** 114–124

Chamberlain, G (1995) *Gynaecology*. Edward Arnold, London

Clarke, A, Black, N and Rowe, P (1995) Indications for the outcome of total abdominal hysterectomy for benign disease: a prospective cohort study. *British Journal of Obstetrics and Gynaecology* **102** 611–620

Hung, P (1992) Preoperative fasting of patients undergoing elective surgery. *British Journal of Nursing* **1**(6) 286–287

Jester, R and Williams, S (1999) Preoperative fasting: putting research into practice. *Nursing Standard* **13**(39) 33–35

Jordan, J A (1989) *Controversies in Gynaecological Oncology*. RCOG, London

Johnson, S (2004) In Whittaker, N (ed) *Disorders and Interventions*. Palgrave, Basingstoke

Kurman, R, Norris, H and Wilkinson, E (1992) *Tumours of the Cervix, Vagina and Vulva*, Vol 4. Armed Forces Institute of Pathology, Washington DC

Lee, K R and Flynn, C E (2000) Early invasive adenocarcinoma of the cervix. *Cancer* **89** 1048–1055

Maltby, J (1993) New guidelines for preoperative fasting. *Canadian Journal of Anaesthesia* **40**(5) 113–117

Namnoun, A B, Gehlbach, D, Hickman, T, Rock, J A and Goodman, S B (1995) Incidence of symptom recurrence after hysterectomy for endometriosis. *Fertility and Sterility* **64** 898–902

O'Callaghan, N (2002) Preoperative fasting. *Nursing Standard* **16**(36) 33–37

Rosevear, S (2002) *Handbook of Gynaecological Management*. Blackwell Science, Oxford

Scottish Hysteroscopy Audit Group (1995) A Scottish audit of hysteroscopic surgery for menorrhagia: complications and follow-up. *British Journal of Obstetrics and Gynaecology* **102** 249–254

Thomas, G M (2000) Concurrent chemotherapy and radiation for locally advanced cervical cancer: the new standard of care. *Seminars in Radiation Oncology* **10** 44–50

Wilson, P D and Bourcler, A (1999) Conservative management in women. In Abrams, P (ed) *Incontinence*. DoH Publication, London

Wyeth UK (2000) *Hysterectomy and Oophorectomy*. http://www.wyeth.co.uk/

Wyeth UK (2002) *The Menopause and The Facts*. http://www.wyeth.co.uk/

Useful addresses

John Wyeth & Brother Ltd
Taplow
Maidenhead
Berkshire
SL6 0PH

British Association for Counselling (BAC)
1 Regent Place
Rugby
CV21 2PJ

The West London Gynaecological Cancer Centre
Queen Charlotte's and Chelsea Hospital
Du Cane Road
London
W12 0HS

Cancer Research UK
Centre for Epidemiology
Wolfson Institute of Preventive Medicine
Charterhouse Square
London
EC1M 6BQ

Useful websites

Gynaesurgeon.co.uk
http://www.gynaesurgeon.co.uk/

British Association for Sexual and Relationship Therapy
http://www.basrt.org.uk/

Family Planning Association
http://www.fpa.org.uk/

CHAPTER 7

Stress urinary incontinence

Introduction

This chapter deals mainly with stress urinary incontinence in women, its predisposing factors, investigations into its causes and the role of the multidisciplinary team in managing this distressing problem.

The anatomical proximity of the urinary bladder and urethra to the female genital tract means that, in many circumstances, pathological conditions that occur in one system impact upon, or involve the anatomy or physiology of, the other. Whilst there are a number of urinary tract problems that are associated with the female reproductive tract (and there are similar genito-urinary system-related problems in males), stress incontinence in women is more common than in men and in 2000 the Department of Health (DoH) issued guidance on establishing integrated continence services (DoH 2000) which became mandatory for the elderly from April 2004 (DoH 2001).

Readers whose knowledge of the anatomy of the female urinary tract and the physiology of micturition is unclear should consult Richardson (2003) for an excellent description.

Urinary incontinence may arise from a number of lower urinary tract anatomical or physiological impairments and can be appropriately diagnosed by:

◇ History taken from the affected woman. History takers should always be aware of the embarrassment that this might cause the historian and listen carefully to the woman's account of the problem(s).

◇ Signs that the doctor observes during the examination.

◇ Results of urodynamic studies (Abrams *et al* 2002).

In order for continence to be maintained:

◇ The nervous system must be intact and have appropriate reflex activity.

◇ The pelvic floor muscles and urethral sphincters need to be effective.

◇ The person must be sufficiently mobile and orientated to reach toilet facilities.

◇ There must be determination to be continent.

Types of incontinence

◇ Urge incontinence – the sudden compelling need to pass urine that is difficult to defer and results in involuntary leakage. This is sometimes related to specific activities such as putting the key in the door and anticipating that the journey to the toilet is short. It would appear that there is almost a 'conditioned reflex' in some women, since if leakage has occurred on one such occasion, it is likely to be repeated in a similar situation on subsequent occasions (McGrother *et al* 2001).

◇ Nocturnal enuresis – involuntarily passing urine whilst asleep.

◇ Continuous urinary incontinence – leakage is involuntary and continuous.

◇ Detrusor overactivity/instability – characterised by a number of symptoms caused by the detrusor muscle of the bladder contracting spontaneously or upon provocation whilst the woman is attempting to withhold micturition.

◇ Genuine stress urinary incontinence – when the pressure within the bladder exceeds the maximum urethral closure pressure in the absence of detrusor activity, urine involuntarily escapes, causing much distress.

There are other types of urinary incontinence, all of which cause varying degrees of torment, anxiety and embarrassment which are not easily spoken of in general conversation.

Stress urinary incontinence (SUI) is a very common condition, having been reported by 16.8% of women in a study by Hunskaar *et al* (2002), and Rothbarth *et al* (2001) talk of the intolerance of western society to even discuss the topic due to its severely debilitating effect upon the quality of life.

Reported prevalence varies between research findings due to different methods of collecting data and the sensitive nature of the questions that need to be put to respondents. McGrother *et al* (2001) reported up to 30% of the population suffering from urinary leakage, with up to 12% of those perceiving it to be problematic.

From the Hunskaar *et al* (2002) research, involving 6,500 UK households, it was established that 4,000,000 women experience SUI, and whilst there is an increase in urinary incontinence with age generally, Hannested *et al* (2000) found that there are peaks in incidence amongst females in the 45–55 years age group and again in those over 70 years. Rosevear (2002) asserts that SUI accounts for 49% of all types of urinary incontinence.

When women seek advice for SUI there is an initial sensitive history-taking process which will usually indicate the next most appropriate investigatory steps.

A physical examination is needed to rule out such factors as pelvic organ prolapse, faecal impaction and previously undiagnosed anatomical abnormality. At this stage a range of procedures, according to early findings, will be arranged to complete the assessment of the problem.

◇ Urinalysis is performed to exclude infection or undiagnosed diabetes mellitus (Shah and Leach 2001). A midstream specimen should be obtained for accurate assessment.

◇ Urine cytology should be performed if symptoms of incontinence with haematuria coexist. This will assist with the exclusion of malignancy of the urinary tract (Shah and Leach 2001).

◇ The patient should be asked to maintain a 'voiding' diary showing frequency and times of micturition and volumes of urine passed – pad tests may be required.

On completion of the above, basic urodynamic investigations involving a number of techniques aimed at monitoring urine flow, bladder muscle contraction and renal function may be ordered. These include:

◇ Uroflowmetry – a non-invasive investigation involving urinating onto a flowmeter which calculates various aspects of volume and rate of flow. It produces a graphical representation of the woman's urinary tract function over a period of time.

◇ Cystometry – a method by which bladder pressure and volume relationship is calculated, indicating the extent of detrusor muscle activity, bladder sensitivity and capacity.

◇ Videocystourethroscopy – the bladder is filled with a radio-opaque medium which can clarify the anatomy of the organ and identify some irregularity of function.

◇ Cystourethroscopy – the bladder and urethra are visualised via a cystoscope and abnormalities such as renal calculi and local tumours can be located. Biopsy of tissue can be performed at the same time.

◇ Intravenous pyelography – a specialised contrast medium X-ray that allows visualisation of the kidneys and can show some types of dysfunction, renal calculi, obstructions and anatomical abnormalities.

◇ Urethral pressure profiltrometry – a test that can demonstrate urine outflow obstruction or failure of the sphincter muscles.

◇ Ultrasound – a useful investigation that is non-invasive and can identify renal calculi and bladder tumours, the anatomy of the bladder and possible ureteric problems.

Once a definite cause has been found, appropriate treatment can be initiated, which, depending upon the cause, general health and wishes of the patient, may be conservative or via surgical intervention.

Conservative therapy is considered when the patient is unfit for or refuses surgery or has not completed her family, or where there are severe detrusor instability/voiding problems. Non-surgical therapy may be in the form of one or several of the following:

◇ Pelvic floor exercises. Theses were introduced in the 1940s by Kegel (1948) and became a popular treatment for SUI. Haslam (2003) advocates exercises that involve the entire abdomino-pelvic cavity in order to improve the strength, power endurance and functionality of the associated muscles. The Royal College of Obstetricians and Gynaecologists (2002) recommends that exercises should continue for up to 20 weeks to achieve the desired result, and only then be referred for possible surgery.

◇ Devices. A number of transvaginal devices have been introduced, such as cones which are weighted and should be inserted into the vagina and held there for 15 minutes, 4 times each day. The weight of the cone is increased as pelvic floor strength improves. Electrical stimulation of the pelvic floor muscles with the use of intravaginal, extravaginal or anal plug electrodes helps some women to overcome SUI if the cones are ineffective.

◇ Drugs. Antibiotics may be prescribed for urinary tract infection and some women may require regular laxatives and drugs to ease the pain of haemorrhoids if either constipation or haemorrhoids contribute to the problem. Phenylpropanolamine, once considered to be very effective as a management drug in the treatment of SUI, has been withdrawn due to the risk of inducing stroke (McPherson and Waller 2003). Norton (2002) found duloxetine to be effective in doses of 20–80 mg daily and safe to use in SUI. This drug is due to become available in 2005. Oestrogen therapy has been found to help some peri- and post-menopausal women (Andersson and Appel 1999).

Matharu *et al* (2004) in their large study, found the combination of pelvic floor exercises and anticholinergic drugs to be effective in many SUI sufferers.

Currently there are no medications available in the *Nurse Prescribers' Formulary* for the treatment of detrusor overactivity and SUI; however, specialist continence advisory nurses can supply anticholinergics, antibiotics and oestrogen cream according to their group protocol.

Surgical management

This has many forms depending upon the main underlying problem, the most widely utilised procedure currently being colposuspension. In the absence of previous surgery, Jarvis (1994) showed an objective cure rate of nearly 90%. The intervention involves an abdominal suprapubic incision with mobilisation of the bladder neck and its elevation by attaching sutures from either side to the ileopectineal or inguinopectineal ligament.

Sling procedures have been used to support the bladder neck and proximal urethra with short-term cure rates similar to colposuspension (Jarvis 1994).

A recently introduced procedure, the 'tension-free vaginal tape' (TVT) has been gaining popularity (NICE 2003) and because it may be carried out using minimal access procedure, local or regional anaesthesia and a short hospital stay (some units manage TVT surgery as a day case procedure), it has several advantages over colposuspension. Nilsson *et al* (2001) reported an 85% objective cure rate following TVT.

Procedure

A small incision is made in the vagina and a permanent tape is introduced to sit under the urethra. Two small (1 cm) incisions are made above the pubic bone through which the tape is withdrawn. As the patient is awake, she can advise the surgeon when adjustments to the tape are made as to which degree of tension is the most comfortable.

The patient is asked to cough so that any leakage can be assessed and a cystoscopy confirms the correct placement of the tape. The abrasive nature of the tape maintains its position.

Serious post-operative problems are rare, but no surgery is without risk and the main complications according to findings by Smith (2000) are:

⬦ Up to 5% of patients experience post-operative voiding difficulties, necessitating catheter insertion.
⬦ 5–10% of patients experience bladder irritability post-operatively.
⬦ 1–5% of women develop urinary tract infection.
⬦ There is a 1% risk of wound infection.

A slight risk of the tape becoming infected or rejected was also reported in this study.

Nursing care input is minimal, as most women are able to return to their pre-operative independent situation within a few hours of the treatment. Whilst this intervention requires longer-term evaluation, the limited morbidity associated with it and the reduced length of hospital stay has potentially huge benefits for both the patient and the National Health Service.

There are other surgical treatments but they do not compare favourably with the above.

Pregnancy and childbirth are acknowledged to be major contributory factors to SUI and it is most important that the midwife encourages pregnant and post-partum women to undertake appropriate pelvic floor exercises to avoid later incontinence.

Obesity, smoking and the menopause have all been implicated (McGrother 2001) and nurses have a health promotion role in relation to these issues.

Conclusion

The high prevalence of SUI in women is due to their anatomical vulnerability, reproductive capacity and hormonal changes. Appropriate assessment and management of urinary incontinence will improve the quality of life for females with this distressing and depressing condition.

Assessment techniques should be meticulously followed in order to determine which steps to take for each individual, commencing with the least invasive and most conservative interventions, offered by competent, knowledgeable and compassionate health professionals.

As medicine is continually striving to advance and many nurses are increasingly accepting roles formerly assigned to junior doctors, it is likely that specialist continence nurse practitioners will be able to prescribe appropriate medications for patients seeking their help. All health care professionals should be able to offer accurate advice to their clients regarding appropriate treatment for incontinence problems.

For some women conservative treatment will be either inappropriate or ineffective, and further investigations will be required prior to more invasive techniques. There will always be women for whom surgery is the most appropriate course of action, and these options must be fully discussed between doctor and patient.

In the case of either a conservative or surgical therapeutic approach the patient should be aware that a cure is not always achievable, but she should expect significant improvement in symptoms.

References

Abrams, P, Cardoza, L and Fall, M (2002) The standardisation of terminology of lower urinary tract function: report from the standardisation committee of the International Continence Society. *Neurological Urodynamics* **21** 167–178

Andersson, K E and Appell, R (1999) Pharmacological treatments of urinary incontinence. In Abrams, P (ed) *Incontinence, 1st International Consultation on Incontinence*. Plymbridge Distributors Ltd, Plymouth

Department of Health (2000) *Good Practice in Continence Services*. DoH, London

Department of Health (2001) *National Service Framework for Older People*. DoH, London

Hannested, Y S, Rortveit, G, Sandvik, H and Hunskaar S (2000) A community-based epidemiological survey of female incontinence: the Norwegian EPICONT study. *Journal of Clinical Epidemiology* **53**(11) 1150–1157

Haslam, J (2003) Pelvic floor muscle exercises. *Nursing Times* **99**(1) 54–55

Hunskaar, S, Lose, G and Viktrup, L (2002) Prevalence of stress urinary incontinence in women in four European countries. *Non discussion poster 257.* International Continence Society Annual Meeting, Heidelberg

Jarvis, G J (1994) Surgery for genuine stress incontinence. *British Journal of Obstetrics and Gynaecology* **101** 371–374

Kegel, A (1948) Progressive resistance exercises in the functional restoration of the perineal muscles. *American Journal of Obstetrics and Gynaecology* **36**(2) 238–248

Matharu, G, Assassa, R P and Williams, K S (2004) Continence nurse treatment of women's urinary symptoms. *British Journal of Nursing* **13**(3) 140–143

McGrother, C W, Shaw, C and Perry, S (2001) *Textbook of Female Urology and Urogynaecology*. Isis Medical Media, Oxford

McPherson, A and Waller, D (eds) (2003) *Women's Health*. Oxford University Press, Oxford

NICE (2003) *Guidance on the use of Tension-Free Vaginal Tape (Gynaecare TVT) for Stress Incontinence*. NICE, London

Nilsson, C, Kuuva, N and Falconer, C (2001) Long-term results of the Tension-Free Vaginal Tape (TVT) for surgical treatment of female stress urinary incontinence. *International Urogynaecological Journal of Pelvic Floor Dysfunction* **12**(Supplement 21) S5–S8

Norton, P A (2002) Duloxetine versus placebo in the treatment of stress incontinence. *American Journal of Obstetrics and Gynaecology* **187**(1) 40–48

Royal College of Obstetricians and Gynaecologists (2002) *42nd Study Group on Incontinence in Women*. RCOG Press, London

Richardson, M (2003) The physiology of micturition. *Nursing Times* **99**(29) 46–48

Rosevear, S (2002) *Handbook of Gynaecological Management*. Blackwell Science, Oxford.

Rothbarth, J, Bemelman, W A and Willhelmus, J H (2001) What is the impact of incontinence on the quality of life? *Diseases of the Colon and Rectum* **39** 860–840

Shah, J and Leach, G (2001) *Urinary Continence.* Health Press, Oxford

Smith, T (2000) Colposcopy. *Nursing Standard* **15**(4) 47

Conclusion

In the preceding chapters, common female reproductive tract functions and dysfunctions have been addressed and, where appropriate, associated legal and professional issues have been discussed. Nurses *must* always be aware of public opinion and how this influences the profession and the law.

Medical and nursing knowledge advances at an increasingly rapid rate, and whilst no professional can be completely aware of every approaching change, it is important that they do know how to access the current information that is likely to affect their day-to-day professional lives and decision-making.

The nursing profession is largely female dominated and the issues outlined in these chapters are commonly encountered by women with gynaecological health problems. The general public has expectations that, when a nurse is approached about a health care issue, s/he will be able to provide a satisfactory answer.

This is particularly true of those very personal, intimate details and subjects that a woman is unlikely to discuss openly and for which she may have to summon up a great deal of courage – even to present to a nurse.

It is incumbent upon all nurses, therefore, to have a reasonable knowledge of the anatomy and physiology of the female reproductive system and the disorders that are potentially problematic, several of which are likely to prompt women to consult nurses regarding investigations that may be arranged and therapeutic interventions that might be organised together with probable outcomes – many of which might subsequently require a great deal of thought by the woman and her partner, depending upon the prevailing condition.

The role of the nurse in gynaecological care is multifactorial and includes the need to maintain confidentiality, to promote the patient's confidence in the National Health Service care delivery, to provide health education and holistic health in the physical, psychological, social and spiritual spheres, and always to act in the best interests of the patient.

Index